Ethical Practice in Forensic Psychology

Ethical Practice
in Forensic Psychology

A Systematic Model for
Decision Making

Shane S. Bush, Mary A. Connell, and Robert L. Denney

AMERICAN PSYCHOLOGICAL ASSOCIATION • WASHINGTON, DC

Published by
American Psychological Association
750 First Street, NE
Washington, DC 20002
www.apa.org

To order
APA Order Department
P.O. Box 92984
Washington, DC 20090-2984
Tel: (800) 374-2721
Direct: (202) 336-5510
Fax: (202) 336-5502
TDD/TTY: (202) 336-6123
Online: www.apa.org/books/
E-mail: order@apa.org

In the U.K., Europe, Africa, and the Middle East, copies may be ordered from
American Psychological Association
3 Henrietta Street
Covent Garden, London
WC2E 8LU England

Typeset in Goudy by World Composition Services, Inc., Sterling, VA

Printer: Book-mart Press, Inc., North Bergen, NJ
Cover Designer: Mercury Publishing Services, Rockville, MD
Technical/Production Editor: Devon Bourexis

The opinions and statements published are the responsibility of the authors, and such opinions and statements do not necessarily represent the policies of the American Psychological Association.

Library of Congress Cataloging-in-Publication Data

Bush, Shane S., 1965-
   Ethical practice in forensic psychology : a systematic model for decision making / Shane S. Bush, Mary A. Connell, Robert L. Denney.— 1st ed.
      p. cm.
   Includes bibliographical references and indexes.
   ISBN 1-59147-395-0
   1. Forensic psychology—Moral and ethical aspects. 2. Forensic psychologists—Professional ethics. 3. Forensic psychology—Practice. I. Connell, Mary A. II. Denney, Robert L. III. Title.

RA1148.B86 2006
174.2′9415—dc22
                                                                              2005034198

British Library Cataloguing-in
A CIP record is available from

Printed in the United States of A
First Edition

To psychologists working in forensic settings who, faced with complex
ethical situations and potential incentives for ethical misconduct,
nevertheless aspire to the highest standards of ethical practice.

IMPORTANT NOTICE

The statements and opinions published in this book are the responsibility of the authors. Such opinions and statements do not represent official policies, standards, guidelines, or ethical mandates of the American Psychological Association (APA), APA's Ethics Committee or Office of Ethics, or any other APA governance group or staff. Statements made in this book neither add to nor reduce requirements of the APA "Ethical Principles of Psychologists and Code of Conduct" (2002), hereinafter referred to as the APA Ethics Code or the Ethics Code, nor can they be viewed as a definitive source of the meaning of the Ethics Code Standards or their application to particular situations. Each ethics committee or other relevant body must interpret and apply the Ethics Code as it believes proper, given all the circumstances. Any information in this book involving legal and ethical issues should not be used as a substitute for obtaining personal legal and/or ethical advice and consultation prior to making decisions regarding individual circumstances.

CONTENTS

PREFACE

As psychologists practicing in various forensic contexts, we have strong personal commitments to establishing and maintaining high standards of ethical practice. Our individual pursuits and studies of ethical principles, standards, guidelines, and other resources led us in a variety of directions and resulted in a rather piecemeal approach to understanding appropriate conduct. Our primary reason for writing this book was to bring together many of the key ethical concepts and resources that we have found valuable and to apply them to forensic psychology.

We are indebted to the many authors who have previously written about psychological ethics, and we are particularly grateful to those who have explored ethical issues in forensic psychology and related psychological specialties; without their work, this book would not have been possible. We are appreciative of the many colleagues with whom we have discussed cases and debated controversial ethical issues; the development and application of professional ethics is an evolving process, and such discussions keep the evolution alive. We are grateful to the legal system for allowing us to contribute to what we hope are just determinations and quality consultative and clinical services.

Ethical Practice
in Forensic Psychology

INTRODUCTION

Thoughts of forensic involvement evoke mixed reactions from psychologists. Some psychologists find forensic practice very appealing; others are extremely frightened by the prospect of being involved in the legal system; and still others fall somewhere in between. Although psychologists who are drawn to forensic activities will undoubtedly face the unique ethical challenges associated with forensic practice, many psychologists with little or no interest in professional legal involvement will nevertheless find themselves thrust into the adversarial process and confronting ethical challenges for which they are not adequately prepared. This book is designed to help prepare career forensic psychologists, forensic psychology students and trainees, and clinical practitioners who inadvertently become involved in forensic matters to successfully avoid and negotiate ethical challenges.

Although this book is, to our knowledge, the first to be solely devoted to ethical issues in forensic psychology, much of the content is compiled from the seminal work of forensic psychology experts who have written and presented before. Throughout the book, we have summarized, integrated, and referenced the works of many psychologists who have laid, and continue to build upon, the foundation of ethical practice in forensic psychology. It is only because of these psychologists and their innovative works that this book was possible.

Unanimous agreement about optimal ethical practices in forensic psychology is lacking, even among those who frequently write and present on the topic. However, themes emerge in the literature that seem to offer general guidance to psychologists who are wishing to prevent, or struggling to negotiate, ethical dilemmas in forensic practice. We have attempted to bring these themes to the reader so that they can be incorporated into daily practices.

It has been said that ethics papers and books raise more questions than they answer (Goodman, 1998). The extent to which that is true of this text, like most ethical matters, depends on what questions are asked. If one asks "What are the ethical issues of greatest concern in forensic psychology?" or "What model can one follow to negotiate ethical challenges in forensic psychology?" then this text will likely provide the answers sought. In contrast, if one asks for guidance to an ethical dilemma, such as, "What should I do when I'm asked to have my evaluation of an examinee taped?" then the information provided may be less specific than desired.

Psychologists involved in forensic practice perform widely ranging professional services in extremely varied settings with a broad spectrum of clients, examinees, and patients. As a result, the specific ethical questions with which psychologists struggle do not lend themselves to cookbook answers that will apply to everyone. Nevertheless, by clarifying the ethical issues and providing a format that psychologists can use to find solutions that are applicable to their specific situations, this text may be of value.

We believe that psychologists involved in forensic practice activities require two things to avoid or negotiate ethical misconduct: (a) a personal commitment to maintaining the highest standards of ethical practice and (b) the information and tools needed to achieve and maintain ethical practice. This book is intended to contribute to the second of the two; that is, to be a source of information and provide some of the tools needed to achieve and maintain ethical practice. Although the wide variety of potential forensic activities for psychologists prohibits exhaustive coverage of issues and practices, we hope that readers will find the book beneficial for enhancing sensitivity to ethical concerns and problem-solving strategies.

The practice of psychology in forensic contexts can be both rewarding and challenging, and the successful negotiation of the challenges can itself be rewarding. The purpose of this book is to provide information that may better position psychologists engaged in forensic practice activities to prevent and negotiate ethical challenges. This book is intended to serve as a text for forensic psychology students, trainees, and practitioners and as a reference guide for all psychologists anticipating involvement in, or unexpectedly thrust into, a legal matter.

UNDERSTANDING, ADOPTING, AND APPLYING PROFESSIONAL ETHICS

Psychologists have at their disposal a variety of ethics resources for determining appropriate courses of professional behavior. The view psychologists take of professional ethics will considerably influence their professional behavior. Those who view ethics solely as a means of enforcing minimal standards of practice fail to appreciate that professional ethics, including the American Psychological Association's (APA) "Ethical Principles of Psychologists and Code of Conduct," (hereinafter APA Ethics Code or Ethics Code; 2002; http://www.apa.org/ethics/code2002.html; see also the appendix at the end of this book), represents an attempt to translate core ethical principles and their underlying human values into operationally defined guidelines for psychologists. Professional codes of ethics, despite their essential contribution for guiding behavior, need not always be the final word on how an issue should best be resolved.

Forensic psychologists have an obligation to the field and to those who are served to not simply be guided by that which is ethically permissible but to seek that which is ethically preferable. The extra steps required to determine ethically preferable courses of action and to pursue such courses of action may require additional effort in the short term, but from that effort will come greater benefits to forensic psychology and the public in the long run. As Knapp and VandeCreek (2003) stated, "The standards in the Ethics Code are designed only to address egregious misconduct. Psychologists who wish to perform at a higher level of skill need to supplement their ethics education with sources beyond the Ethics Code" (p. 16).

With this book we strive to present and integrate the principles and standards provided in the APA Ethics Code with many of the other guidelines that have relevance to forensic practice. This book is intended to provide forensic psychology students and trainees and practicing psychologists who have little forensic involvement with the ability to apply appropriate professional resources to ethical challenges associated with specific practice activities. In addition, by reviewing relevant sections of the book as needed, career forensic psychologists may achieve greater understanding of challenging ethical issues and increased ease of ethical problem solving.

FORMAT OF THE BOOK

There are a number of possible ways to organize a forensic psychology ethics book, including organizing the material around (a) the steps in the evaluation process, such as the referral, data collection, and so on; (b) forensic topics areas, such as civil litigation and criminal litigation; (c) the relevant ethical principles; or (d) threats to the validity of the data or the opinions provided, such as inadequate competence and compromised objectivity. The first option was chosen for this text. Our reason for choosing to organize the material around the steps in the evaluation process is that it provides clear reference points for practicing psychologists who are facing ethical challenges. Although practitioners may not always be immediately aware of the relevant ethical principles or the underlying threats to the validity of data or opinions, they do know the practice activity in which they or their colleagues are engaging. Thus, organization along these lines facilitates reference to the material that is most relevant at a given time. The material was not organized according to forensic topic areas because the considerable overlap of relevant ethical issues across topic areas would require excessive redundancy in the coverage of material. The emphasis on the evaluation process is not meant to minimize the importance of ethics for the many nonevaluation forensic activities (e.g., treatment, trial consultation) in which psychologists engage; it simply reflects an element of practice that we have found to be a focus for many forensic psychologists. We hope that the ethical issues examined and the decision-making process described in the context of the forensic evaluation can be readily applied to a broad range of forensic practice activities.

Following this introduction, chapters 2 through 6 examine the various components of the forensic evaluation process, beginning with the referral and ending with testimony. Although much of the information applies to psychologists working in forensic treatment settings and as trial consultants, the book is structured primarily around the forensic evaluation. Case illustrations are provided to demonstrate application of the issues examined and the ethical decision-making process. Case illustrations cover three broad topic areas: personal injury litigation, criminal litigation, and child and family law. Chapter 7 covers the ethical challenges inherent in addressing ethical misconduct by colleagues doing forensic work. Forensic psychologists are likely exposed to more of the work of colleagues than are psychologists in any other specialty area. That exposure, combined with the natural emotional reactions and the potential for bias that may emerge in adversarial situations, contributes to a context in which allegations of ethical misconduct may abound. This raises a need for attention to be given to the sensitive topic of responding to apparent ethical misconduct by forensic psychology colleagues. The Afterword offers concluding remarks, with an emphasis on the personal commitment needed by forensic psychologists for ethical conduct to be possible.

The book includes "excerpts" from fictional psychological and neuropsychological reports. These excerpts were created by the authors and represent an amalgam of reports by numerous psychologists that the authors reviewed over the years. Similarly, the case illustrations provided in the book were created by the authors and represent an integration of scenarios either encountered in practice or imagined by the authors. Despite any unintended similarities, the excerpts and case illustrations do not represent the reports or practice of any given psychologist.

1

THE INTERFACE OF LAW AND PSYCHOLOGY: AN OVERVIEW

The profession of psychology has much to offer the legal system and those with possible or clearly identified psychological difficulties who find themselves negotiating the legal system. As a result, forensic psychology has emerged as a distinct specialty area within the broader field of psychology. *Forensic psychology* includes both scholarly and applied activities and represents the intersection of clinical and experimental psychology and the law (Heilbrun, 2001). The clinical and experimental forensic arenas are themselves composed of diverse psychological specialties, such as counseling, developmental, and social psychology. Thus, forensic psychologists may have multiple professional identities representing both their primary areas of training and experience and their subsequent application of their knowledge and skills to forensic matters.

In addition to psychologists who pursue professional involvement in the legal system, some clinicians inadvertently find themselves involved in the legal matters of their patients. Involvement of the clinician may be either requested or required. For example, a neuropsychologist may be subpoenaed to testify about the evaluation findings of a patient who sustained a traumatic brain injury in a motor vehicle accident. Understanding the professional, ethical, and legal issues involved in such situations is necessary for successful performance of one's responsibilities.

Because of the varied contexts in which forensic psychologists practice, there will likely be exceptions to many of the topics examined in this text. Nevertheless, an increased understanding of the ethical issues that pertain to forensic psychology in general will assist psychologists in all forensic contexts to better serve those with whom they interact professionally. For the purposes of this text, the term *forensic psychologist* is used broadly to refer to those psychologists who perform forensic activities or work in forensic settings; it is not used solely to denote those with specialized training or board certification in forensic psychology.

FORENSIC PSYCHOLOGY IN CIVIL AND CRIMINAL CONTEXTS

Psychologists serve the justice system in a variety of contexts (Blau, 1998; Heilbrun, 2001; Koocher & Keith-Spiegel, 1998; Melton, Petrila, Poythress, & Slobogin, 1997; Walker & Shapiro, 2003). They can be found practicing and conducting research in both civil and criminal legal arenas. Civil law includes matters of family law; administrative proceedings, such as Worker's Compensation; and tort law, such as personal injury litigation. Typically, the purpose of civil law is to assign responsibility for harm and to provide a remedy. However, family law, a type of civil law, differs from other civil matters in several important ways. In family law matters, the court is generally called on to resolve disputes having to do with the following: (a) marital dissolution, where there may or may not be a finding of fault; (b) determinations regarding parenting relationships, such as parenting agreements following divorce, adoption proceedings, or proceedings to terminate parental rights; and (c) matters of juvenile justice that do not fall within the purview of criminal law, owing to the status of the actor as a minor.

In contrast to civil law, criminal law is based on the concept of "moral blameworthiness" (Behnke, Perlin, & Bernstein, 2003). When an individual has been found guilty of a crime, a moral sanction applies, including removal from society if deemed necessary by the court. Criminal law addresses a number of steps in determining the guilt or innocence of a defendant and providing a consequence if the accused is found guilty. Psychological expertise and services can be found across the continuum of criminal law.

In both civil and criminal contexts, psychologists engage in professional activities relevant to a wide range of legal and psychological issues. According to Standard 7-11 of the Criminal Justice Mental Health Standards (American Bar Association [ABA], 1989),

> Mental health and mental retardation professionals serve the adminis-
> tration of criminal justice by offering expert opinions and testimony

within their respective areas of expertise concerning present scientific or clinical knowledge; by evaluating and offering expert opinions and testimony on the mental condition of defendants and witnesses; by providing consultation to the prosecution or defense concerning the conduct of individual cases; and by providing treatment and habilitation for persons charged with or convicted of crimes. Because these roles involve differing and sometimes conflicting obligations and functions, these professionals as well as courts, attorneys, and criminal justice agencies should clarify the nature and limitations of these respective roles.

Forensic Evaluation Services

The forensic psychology evaluation differs considerably from the clinical psychology evaluation. Differences begin with the language used to describe the evaluation. Psychological evaluations performed by practitioners who are hired as independent contractors by third parties, such as disability insurers, attorneys, or the courts, are often referred to as *independent psychological examinations* or *independent medical examinations*. Differences between forensic and clinical evaluations also include the nature of the requested evaluation, which has theoretical and practical implications for the manner in which the task is approached (Denney & Wynkoop, 2000). With forensic evaluation services, context affects (a) the goals of the evaluation, (b) the psychologist's role, (c) the assumptions the psychologist makes about the accuracy of information received from the examinee, (d) alliances formed, and (e) methodology used by the psychologist.

The purpose of a forensic evaluation is to assist the legal decision maker (Melton et al., 1997), who may be a judge, juror, mediator, or other hearing officer. This forensic purpose stands in contrast to the clinician's goal of assisting the patient. Accepting that the psychologist's primary obligation is to the legal decision maker rather than to the examinee may be a difficult transition to make for psychologists who have been clinically trained. However, it is necessary for examining psychologists to understand that the retaining party is the client and that the examinee is neither a patient nor the client of the examining psychologist. Exceptions may exist in forensic treatment settings in which evaluations may be performed to facilitate clinical services rather than to inform legal decisions.

The goal of the psychologist retained to serve as an expert witness is to provide information useful to the trier of fact in its effort to answer a specific legal question, such as the presence or absence of psychological "damages" or competency to stand trial. To achieve this goal, the psychologist assumes the role of seeker of truth and judicial educator (Denney & Wynkoop, 2000; Saks, 1990). The opinions provided are not designed to help the examinee; in some instances, the opinions offered may conflict with the litigant's wishes.

The psychologist retained to serve as an expert witness cannot assume that the information received from the litigant is accurate. Litigants may not even be voluntary participants in the evaluation. The possible outcomes of litigation can create tremendous motivation for the litigant to manipulate the evaluator. It is counterproductive to trust the presentation of such highly invested examinees without verification.

The alliances that a psychologist maintains may differ depending on the context of the service provided. Although a psychologist providing treatment typically forms a therapeutic alliance with the patient, such an alliance with a forensic examinee may not be necessary or appropriate (S. Greenberg & Shuman, 1997). The psychologist retained as an expert witness forms an alliance with the truth. The investment in determining and reporting the truth may make problematic the establishment of rapport between examiner and examinee. Rapport may be misconstrued as an offer of advocacy and may lure the examinee into a level of disclosure that is not in the examinee's best legal interest. A posture of respectful receptivity with an arms-length, or dispassionate, mien may be the most appropriate posture to assume during the examination.

The context in which the evaluation is performed also affects the methodology used by the psychologist. Forensic psychological evaluations require a broader base of information sources than is typical of clinical practice, a base that extends well beyond the self-report of the examinee (Denney & Wynkoop, 2000). In contrast to the urgency that is often required in the provision of clinical evaluation services, psychologists practicing in forensic contexts must take the time necessary to ensure that the broad base of information that is needed (e.g., interviews, observations, records, test data) can be obtained and thoroughly reviewed before conclusions are offered.

The Distinction Between the Roles of Expert Witness and Treating Doctor

The distinction between the roles of treating doctor and forensic psychological expert has been the focus of some discussion in forensic psychology ethics (e.g., J. M. Fisher, Johnson-Greene, & Barth, 2002; S. Greenberg & Shuman, 1997; Iverson, 2000). Both of these roles are subsumed under the first ABA role definition cited earlier, that of "offering expert opinions and testimony concerning present scientific or clinical knowledge" (ABA, 1989, Standard 7-1.1, ¶ 6). In the treatment role, the psychologist may be required to provide records to, or testify before, the court on a legal matter in which the psychological functioning or treatment of a patient may be relevant to the court. In such instances, the psychologist is considered a fact witness,[1] testifying about diagnostic impressions and the facts of the treatment.

Opinions about the clinical interpretation of data are relevant contributions, but the treating therapist rarely has accomplished an arms-length, comprehensive assessment that would lead to defensible opinion on the psycholegal issue. Although there is controversy about whether the treating clinician should offer opinion on the ultimate issue before the court, the treating psychologist must limit opinion to that for which adequate data has been gathered. For example, a therapist might opine about the likely impact of the child patient's visitation with a parent the therapist has never met, if the therapist makes clear the limitations of that opinion (i.e., that it is based only on the child's and possibly other parent's presentation; that the therapist is an advocate for the patient and has not "heard the other side of the story"; that the interpretation of data collected in therapy is more subjective and potentially less reliable than data gathered from a range of sources including objective measures, careful records review, collateral consultation, and so on). Even with such careful statement of these limitations, the therapist testifying about matters before the court must be aware of the potential for the court to misconstrue or misuse the opinion data. The therapist who has risked this misuse of data may find little support in the professional community for offering opinion derived through provision of psychotherapy as an expert evaluation of the forensic issue (S. Greenberg & Shuman, 1997; Heilbrun, 1995, 2001; Melton et al., 1997). The distinction, then, is between being an expert clinician and being a forensic examiner for the purpose of developing an opinion, to be offered in court, on a psycholegal matter. Both may function as experts in the court, and the clinician may be able to provide expert opinion on the clinical data, but generally the clinician has insufficient data to offer an opinion on the matter before the court.

To facilitate clinical treatment, the treating doctor may provide diagnostic impressions prior to performing a complete review of relevant records, interviewing collateral sources of information, conducting thorough psychodiagnostic testing, or otherwise performing an evaluation adequate to answer questions before the court "with a reasonable degree of certainty." In contrast

---

[1] The distinction between *fact witness* and *expert witness*, although common in psychological writings, is not found in the *Federal Rules of Evidence* (FRE; 1975). The FRE (Article VII, Opinions and Expert Testimony) distinguishes only between expert and lay witnesses, and it is the court that makes the determination for any given case. The term *fact witness* is not found in the FRE.

to the clinical role, the forensic psychological expert role requires (a) a review of all materials and completion of all procedures upon which to base an opinion sufficient to withstand judicial scrutiny and (b) an objective and judgmental position that may be impossible for the typically accepting and nonjudgmental clinician to achieve (Shuman & Greenberg, 1998).

The term *treating doctor* has at times been used inappropriately to describe all clinical activities, such as clinical diagnostic evaluations that do not involve remedial intervention or advocacy (Bush, 2004b). Although clinical evaluations are typically performed to facilitate therapy, they are not intended to be therapeutic in and of themselves. Thus, the goals, assumptions, and alliances of the clinical examiner may more closely parallel those of the forensic examiner than those of the treating therapist.

The distinction between *treating doctor* and *expert witness* is limited and is insufficient to understand the forensic roles of psychologists (Bush, 2004b). Heilbrun (2001) described five possible roles for mental health professionals in forensic assessment contexts: clinical or court-appointed evaluator; defense, prosecution, or plaintiff's expert; scientific advisor to the court; consultant; and fact witness. This broad description of roles better reflects the breadth of psychologists' potential professional forensic involvement.

Blurring of Professional, Clinical, and Forensic Roles

The role held by the psychologist has implications for objectivity and accuracy in the presentation of information to the court and, by extension, the accuracy of judicial determinations (Shuman & Greenberg, 1998). Blurring of professional, clinical, and forensic roles has the strong potential to invoke conflicts of interest that negatively affect one or more of the roles (Shuman & Greenberg, 1998). Psychologists have a responsibility to recognize the potential for conflicts of interest in dual or multiple relationships with parties to a legal proceeding and to seek to minimize their effects (Standards 3.05, Multiple Relationships, and 3.06, Conflict of Interest, of the American Psychological Association's [APA's] Ethics Code, 2002; Specialty Guidelines for Forensic Psychologists [SGFP] IV, Relationships, subsection D, from the Committee on Ethical Guidelines for Forensic Psychologists, 1991). In general, to maximize objectivity, these roles should not be combined in a single case (Denney, 2005; Heilbrun, 2001).

One potential exception to the principle of avoiding dual relationships may be seen in the psychologist who transitions from the role of examiner to that of trial consultant after all evaluation-related responsibilities have been completed. For example, a psychologist who is retained by a criminal defense attorney to conduct an evaluation and provide verbal feedback, who is asked to not write a report, and who will not later testify might appropriately transition to the role of consultant. The psychologist in this scenario will have completed the role of examiner and will no longer be required to maintain impartiality.

Some forensic mental health professionals want to have it both ways, to be healers and to serve the adversary system (Stone, 1984). L. R. Greenberg and Gould (2001) took the position that, in some situations, psychologists may ethically have it both ways. They described a "hybrid role" in which the treating psychologist whose patients have impending or ongoing litigation should be sensitive to the unique experiences and needs of such patients, should be aware that the litigation will likely impact the therapy, and should possess many of the practice-related traits of the forensic examiner, while maintaining firm limits regarding the nature of the opinion testimony provided (L. R. Greenberg & Gould, 2001). As these researchers described, although the treating psychologist may provide opinions regarding diagnosis, treatment, and prognosis, "the treating expert generally declines to express opinions on psycholegal issues (e.g., custody recommendations and parental capacity)" (p. 477). When overlapping or multiple roles are adopted, it is how the overlap is managed that distinguishes ethical conduct from misconduct.

Although psychologists may define the factors that compose a forensic psychological evaluation and the factors that characterize a competent expert witness, it is ultimately the court that determines what evidence will be allowed and who will be considered an expert in a particular case. The adversarial system is designed to provide the checks and balances for determining the adequacy (relevance and reliability) of the psychologist's work product. It is the psychological sophistication of the attorneys, trial consultants, and trier of fact involved in the case that will determine the effectiveness of the adversarial system for cases in which psychological functioning is at issue. It is the responsibility of the psychologist to provide education to those who do not appreciate the threats to impartiality and to attempt to maintain clear distinctions in professional roles.

THE ADVERSARIAL ENVIRONMENT

Expert witnesses play a prominent role in the U.S. litigation process (Crown, Fingerhut, & Lowenthal, 2003); however, the adversarial nature of the U.S. legal system presents unique challenges for psychologists. A primary issue that is unique to many forensic situations is that the practitioner's opinions may be challenged or questioned. The "opponent" mounting this challenge is an individual or team of individuals who question the practitioner's methods, opinions, and qualifications. A psychologist retained by the defense attorney in a civil case or by the prosecution in a criminal case to provide an "independent" opinion will be seen by some examinees as an opponent, a perception that may alter the examinee's behavior during the exam. The perception of the psychologist as an opponent leads to many of the ethical dilemmas that are faced by forensic psychologists.

The adversarial environment may also pit psychologists against those who have retained their services. The attorney who has retained a psychologist to perform an evaluation has an allegiance to the client and must diligently advocate for the client. In contrast, the examining psychologist has a responsibility to remain objective. Although retained by the attorney, the psychologist has an allegiance to the court. This inherent clash between the attorney as advocate and the expert witness, whose single most important obligation is to approach each question with independence and objectivity (Crown et al., 2003; Lubet, 1999), is also a source of ethical conflict for psychologists.

Psychologists are not always adequately prepared by their education and predoctoral training for these challenges. Thus, for many psychologists, the transition from the classroom or clinical setting to a forensic environment may involve a substantial paradigm shift and a corresponding struggle with the ethical, moral, and legal issues involved (Martelli, Bush, & Zasler, 2003). The most logical approach to both advancing ethical practice and availing the legal system of one's expertise may be to develop an increased sensitivity to the disparities between conflicting interests and ethics.

THE NEED FOR INFORMATION ON ETHICS IN FORENSIC PSYCHOLOGY

The pulls to sacrifice objectivity, the differences between clinical and forensic activities, and the enticement to step beyond the boundaries of one's competence all provide opportunities for ethical misconduct. Particularly in today's health care environment, in which shrinking reimbursement for services is often coupled with increased time-consuming clerical requirements, the lure of higher fees for one's services may draw inadequately prepared clinicians into professionally dangerous waters. Similarly, financial incentives may lead even the most qualified forensic psychologist into unethical behaviors that are harmful to the retaining party, examinee, legal system, and profession of psychology. An awareness of the common ethical challenges in forensic psychology can help psychologists examine their own practices and the practices of their colleagues.

APPLYING GENERAL BIOETHICAL PRINCIPLES
IN FORENSIC ARENAS

All ethical principles are based on fundamental human values. Values that a society deems important, such as the right to self-determination and the right to quality health care, are applied to specific industries and professions. Beauchamp and Childress (2001) offered a model of biomedical ethics that has been widely adopted by writers in a variety of health care specialties, including psychology. The model is composed of four basic principles: autonomy, nonmaleficence, beneficence, and justice. Psychologists may recognize the last three principles from the APA Ethics Code. The first principle, autonomy, is also present in the Ethics Code, embedded in General Principle E (Respect for People's Rights and Dignity).

Autonomy refers to self-determination, the ability to make decisions regarding one's life. *Nonmaleficence* is closely related to the Hippocratic Oath: First, do no harm. *Beneficence* takes clinician responsibility a step further by requiring an attempt to promote that which is beneficial to the patient. In health care settings, *justice* typically refers to the equitable distribution of the burdens and benefits of care (Hanson, Guenther, Kerkhoff, & Liss, 2000). Stone (1984) noted that "to many moral philosophers, justice is itself a beneficence" (p. 71). He elaborated as follows:

> Justice is a beneficence to a society of unidentified persons—that is, to the general good. In contrast, the doctor's practical ethical duty is to ease the suffering of particular identified patients. Medicine has not yet solved the problem of how to balance the particular good of the identified patient against the general good of the unidentified masses. We lose our practical ethical guidelines when we try to serve such greater good in the courtroom. (p. 71)

Biomedical ethical principles can be readily applied to most ethical challenges in clinical psychology where the clinician's goal is to help patients, to avoid harm, to respect the wishes of patients regarding their treatment, and to practice in a just and fair manner. However, in an adversarial judicial system, the application of these principles may initially appear to be far more challenging.

In forensic practice, psychologists have a responsibility to respect the rights of examinees and other clients to determine their involvement in psychological services. Examinees participate in independent psychological evaluations more or less of their own accord, albeit at times under the threat of negative consequences should they choose not to participate. In legal contexts, the concepts of "nonmaleficence" and "justice" are closely tied (Martelli et al., 2003). Forensic psychologists have a responsibility to treat examinees with courtesy, dignity, and fairness. Beyond the possibility of invoking emotional reactions to evaluation questions or tasks, practitioners must not bring direct harm to examinees during evaluations. Nevertheless, the results of forensic psychological evaluations and subsequent testimony have the potential to result in considerable negative effects on the lives of examinees. It is the psychologist's responsibility to perform a fair evaluation and to present the findings objectively and dispassionately. The legal decision maker then has the task of ensuring a just outcome. An examinee who believes he or she has been treated fairly and respectfully is less likely to perceive the examiner as being maleficent, even given an unfavorable determination.

For forensic examinations, helping the examinee is not a primary goal of the examiner. Helping the trier of fact to make an appropriate determination taking into account the examinee's cognitive or psychological functioning is a goal. The examinee may or may not benefit from the examination findings. Thus, the principle of beneficence as it relates to forensic psychological services may generally fall within the ambit of the justice system rather than the individual examinee.

Although helping the examinee may not be a primary goal of the examiner, there are nevertheless situations in which the examiner is ethically obligated to assist the examinee. When evidence of maleficence is observed in the course of professional duties, forensic psychologists have a responsibility to report or ameliorate it, with strongest advocacy taken on behalf of the most vulnerable individuals.

Applying bioethical principles in forensic practice can be more complex still. For example, psychologists hired as trial consultants by defense attorneys in civil litigation cases strive to harm the plaintiff's case and, by extension, the plaintiff's financial security. One of the psychologist's roles is to identify errors in the work of the psychologist retained by the plaintiff's attorney, errors that may lead to a decision for the defendant, even if the psychologist believes that the plaintiff actually deserves to win the case. In such a situation, determining whether justice was served may be a difficult thing to do.

The adversarial process is built on the assumption that right will prevail if the responsibilities of all participants are fully discharged. It is not the forensic psychologist's responsibility to ensure retention by the party deserving to prevail. It is the forensic psychologist's responsibility to thoroughly and adequately perform his or her duties; if the resultant outcome favors the "unjust," we believe that the psychologist must forgo a sense of personal responsibility for that injustice. The differences between clinical and forensic contexts notwithstanding, we believe that the Beauchamp and Childress (2001) model is useful in forensic psychology and have chosen to use their model in the more comprehensive decision-making model that is presented later in this chapter.

APPLYING PSYCHOLOGICAL ETHICS IN FORENSIC ARENAS

The 2002 APA Ethics Code is the 10th version of the Ethics Code, and it reflects the continuing evolution and maturation of the profession of psychology. The Ethics Code applies to all psychology specialty areas, including forensic psychology. However, sections of the Ethics Code may hold more or less relevance for various aspects of forensic practice than they do for clinical psychology or other areas of practice. For example, it may be more common to have one's credentials called into question (Standard 2.01, Boundaries of Competence) in forensic practice than it is in clinical practice.

Understanding changes between different versions of the APA Ethics Code that are relevant to forensic practice is essential when determining appropriate professional conduct.[2] Because previous texts addressed the changes to the Ethics Code in some detail (e.g., C. B. Fisher, 2003a; Knapp & VandeCreek, 2003), this section provides only a brief overview, with emphasis on those changes that are most relevant to forensic psychology.

General Principles

The 2002 APA Ethics Code's General Principles reflect increased emphasis on the model of biomedical ethics described by Beauchamp and Childress (2001). This model centers on four ethical principles: autonomy, beneficence, nonmaleficence, and justice. Autonomy, the right to self-determination, remains reflected in General Principle E (Respect for People's Rights and Dignity). Beneficence and nonmaleficence (new General Principle A) were previously reflected in the Ethics Code but now emphasize, in greater detail, the goal of assisting without harming those with whom psychologists work. Justice, a new addition to the Ethics Code, is addressed in General Principle D. The principle of justice emphasizes the right to equality in access to psychological services and in the nature of the services provided. It also emphasizes for psychologists the importance of ensuring that potential biases and limitations of professional competence do not result in unfair practices. The Ethics Code was reduced from six principles

---

[2]For interested readers, comparisons of the two APA Ethics Codes can be found on the APA Ethics Office Web site at http://www.apa.org/ethics/codecompare/html. The comparisons describe which principles and standards were added, deleted, or incorporated into other areas of the Ethics Code.

to five. Prior principles, titled "Competence" and "Social Responsibility," were deleted. Issues of professional competence, on the basis of the underlying principle of nonmaleficence, now compose Standard 2 (Competence). Previous content related to social responsibility was incorporated in the Preamble and Introduction.

Ethical Standards

The elimination of a separate group of standards on forensic activities (Standard 7) is of particular significance and interest to psychologists who are involved in forensic practice. Of the five subsections of Standard 7 in the 1992 APA Ethics Code (APA, 1992), four were deleted, and the content related to role clarification was integrated into Standard 3 (Human Relations) in the 2002 Ethics Code. The purpose of deleting Standard 7 was to eliminate the focus on any one specialty area and to keep the focus of the Ethics Code on issues that are relevant to psychology in general. The Ethics Code Task Force intended to make the Ethics Code as generic as possible (Knapp & VandeCreek, 2003). Nevertheless, forensic activities received emphasis in some sections of the 2002 Ethics Code, including Standards 2.01f, Boundaries of Competence; 9.01a, Bases for Assessments; 9.03c, Informed Consent in Assessments; and 9.10, Explaining Assessment Results. In addition to the Ethical Standards that specifically mention forensic activities, the following changes, outlined in this section and presented in greater detail in subsequent chapters, hold particular relevance for forensic practice.

The manner in which psychologists are to resolve ethical issues was moved from the last standard to the first (Standard 1, Resolving Ethical Issues). This standard is particularly relevant because of the sensitive nature of handling ethical misconduct during the course of litigation. Issues of competence now compose Standard 2 (Competence). The transition of Competence from a General Principle to an Ethical Standard reflects an increased emphasis on the importance of psychologists understanding that attainment of competence is not simply aspirational but is an essential requirement for ethical psychological practice. Attainment of competence in one area of psychology does not imply competence in another. Competence must be established in each area within which forensic psychologists practice and with each population with which forensic psychologists work. Competence must be maintained through continuing education and peer consultation.

Standard 3.10c, Informed Consent, is a new addition to the APA Ethics Code that explains consent obligations when psychological services are court ordered or otherwise mandated. In addition, issues related to informed consent were included, for the first time, in the section on assessment. Standard 9.03, Informed Consent in Assessments, describes the consent process in detail, including exceptions to the need to obtain informed consent. These standards support the obligation of psychologists to attempt to describe to patients and examinees the potential foreseeable uses and implications of treatment records or evaluation results as early in the professional relationship as possible.

Standards addressing multiple relationships (Standards 3.05, Multiple Relationships; 3.06, Conflicts of Interest; and 10.02, Therapy Involving Couples or Families) were clarified in the new APA Ethics Code. Forensic psychologists must refrain from accepting a professional role if it may be reasonably assumed that there is compromised objectivity or some circumstance that negatively affects the psychologist's ability to effectively perform professional activities. In addition, the 2002 Ethics Code indicates that multiple relationships that would not be reasonably expected to interfere with professional behavior or result in harm are not unethical (Standard 3.05a).

The 2002 APA Ethics Code includes an increased emphasis on cultural competency in situations in which it has been determined that such competency is essential for effective service delivery (Standard 2.01b, Boundaries of Competence). The new Ethics Code also emphasizes the importance of sensitivity to the difficulties inherent in providing services when language fluency between psychologist and patient or examinee differs. Standard 9.02b, Use of Assessments, requires psychologists to use assessment instruments for which reliability and validity have been established with members of the population that the examinee represents. Standard 9.02c, also new, requires psychologists to use measures that are appropriate given the examinee's language preference and competence, unless use of an alternative language is relevant to the evaluation. Standard 9.06, Interpreting Assessment Results, states that linguistic and cultural differences must be appropriately considered when interpreting results. Throughout Standard 9, the Ethics Code stresses the importance of describing the limitations of one's interpretations. Standard 9.03, Informed Consent in Assessments, describes the need to obtain informed consent from the examinee regarding the use of an interpreter. Information provided to the examinee includes the possibility that interpretation may result in a degree of imprecision in the evaluation results, and the extent of the imprecision will be greater the more the interpreter and the examinee vary in their dialect or regional nuances. Standard 9.03c also emphasizes the need for psychologists to ensure that interpreters appreciate confidentiality rights and limitations and that they maintain test security.

The 2002 APA Ethics Code includes a significant change to the manner in which psychologists are to handle requests for test data and materials. In the Ethics Code a distinction is made between *test data* and *test materials*. *Test data* (as defined in Standard 9.04a, Release of Test Data) refers to "raw and scaled scores, client/patient responses to test questions or stimuli, and psychologists' notes and recordings concerning client/patient statements and behavior during an examination." Under the 1992 Ethics Code, psychologists were required to refrain from releasing raw data to anyone (other than the patient or client under certain circumstances) not qualified to interpret or appropriately use the data. Under current guidelines, with a client–patient release, psychologists must provide test data to the client–patient or to anyone identified in the release, unless the psychologist believes that "substantial harm or misuse or misrepresentation" (Standard 9.04a) may result. In Standard 9.11, Maintaining Test Security, *test materials* are defined as "manuals, instruments, protocols, and test questions." In contrast to what is required for *test data*, psychologists are required to "make reasonable efforts to maintain the integrity and security of test materials" (Standard 9.11). Standard 9.04a includes as test data those materials that have examinee responses written on them. That is, test materials that must be safeguarded convert to test data that can generally be released (with client consent) once the psychologist or examinee has written responses on them (Behnke, 2003).

The 2002 APA Ethics Code includes a section on record reviews and opinions proffered without the psychologist having examined the subject of the opinion (Standard 9.01c, Bases for Assessments). When an opinion is offered in the absence of an examination, the psychologist must explain the reasons for not conducting an examination and describe the information upon which the decisions and opinions were based, including any limitations inherent in the absence of the examination. Standard 9.01c reflects a departure from the 1992 requirement that, with some exceptions, psychologists perform face-to-face examinations when offering diagnostic or evaluative statements or recommendations, particularly in forensic contexts (APA, 1992 [1992 Standards 2.01, Evaluation, Diagnosis, and Interventions in Professional Context; 7.02b and 7.02c, Forensic Assessments; Knapp & Vandecreek, 2003).

RELATED PROFESSIONAL GUIDELINES

As the "Introduction and Applicability" section of the 2002 APA Ethics Code states, "Psychologists may consider other materials and guidelines that have been adopted or endorsed by scientific and professional psychological organizations" during the process of making decisions about professional behavior. To go a step further, we suggest that forensic psychologists must consider guidelines promulgated within their areas of specialization and appropriately endorsed by recognized organizations leading the field to which they apply. The general nature of the Ethics Code offers a solid foundation for many aspects of forensic practice, but more specific application of ethical principles and acceptable practice parameters is required and can be found in a number of publications from APA and other professional organizations. Table 1.1 provides a summary of some of the available guidelines. Some of these guidelines undergo periodic revision; as a result, psychologists are encouraged to check the Web sites and publications of the sponsoring organizations periodically to ensure that they are in possession of the most recent versions of the documents.

The Specialty Guidelines for Forensic Psychologists: A Brief Overview

The SGFP were prepared by the American Psychology–Law Society (APA's Division 41) and are endorsed by the American Academy of Forensic Psychology (Committee on Ethical Guidelines for Forensic Psychologists, 1991). Although designed to be consistent with the APA Ethics Code, the SGFP were developed to provide more specific guidance to forensic psychologists than was offered in the Ethics Code. The purpose of the SGFP is to improve the quality of forensic psychological service.

The SGFP consist of an introductory section followed by seven topical sections: Purpose and Scope, Responsibility, Competence, Relationships, Confidentiality and Privilege, Methods and Procedures, and Public and Professional Communications. The SGFP provide a useful supplement to the APA Ethics Code. As of this writing, they are undergoing revision and a multiyear approval process. (The most current draft of the SGFP can be found on the American Psychology–Law Society Web site at http://www.ap-ls.org/links/professionalsgfp.html.)

CONSIDERATION OF JURISDICTIONAL LAWS

The Introduction and Applicability section of the APA Ethics Code instructs psychologists to consider applicable laws and psychology board regulations during their ethical decision-making processes. Psychologists should know the source of the jurisdictional regulations that govern their professional conduct, whether it is the Ethics Code, the Canadian Code of Ethics for Psychologists (Canadian Psychological Association, 2000), the Association of State and Provincial Psychology Boards (2005) Code of Conduct, or some other source.

The Health Insurance Portability and Accountability Act

At the federal level, the Health Insurance Portability and Accountability Act (HIPAA; U.S. Department of Health and Human Services [U.S.

TABLE 1.1
Professional Guidelines Relevant to Forensic Psychology

Organization	Year	Title
AACAP	1997a	Practice Parameters for Child Custody Evaluation
	1997b	Practice Parameters for the Forensic Evaluation of Children and Adolescents Who May Have Been Physically or Sexually Abused
AACN	1999	Policy on the Use of Non-Doctoral-Level Personnel in Conducting Clinical Neuropsychological Evaluations
	2001	Policy Statement on the Presence of Third Party Observers in Neuropsychological Assessments
	2003	Official Position of the American Academy of Clinical Neuropsychology on Ethical Complaints Made Against Clinical Neuropsychologists During Adversarial Proceedings
AAP	1999	Guidelines for the Evaluation of the Sexual Abuse of Children: Subject Review
AAPL	1995	Ethical Guidelines for the Practice of Forensic Psychiatry
AERA, APA,* NCME	1999	Standards for Educational and Psychological Testing
AFCC	1994	Model Standards of Practice for Child Custody Evaluation
AMA	1993a	The Insanity Defense in Criminal Trials and Limitations of Psychiatric Testimony
	1993b	Rape Victim Services
	1997	Bonding Programs for Women Prisoners and Their Newborn Children
	1998a	AMA–ABA Statement on Interprofessional Relations for Physicians and Attorneys
	1998b	Guidelines for Due Process
	1999a	Confidentiality Industry-Employed Physicians and Independent Medical Examiners
	1999b	Patient–Physician Relationships in the Context of Work-Related and Independent Medical Examinations
	2000a	Guidelines for Expert Witness
	2000b	Peer Review and Medical Expert Witness Testimony
	2000c	Prison-Based Treatment Programs for Drug Abuse
	2004a	Expert Witness Affirmation
	2004b	Expert Witness Testimony
	2004c	Scientific Status of Refreshing Recollection by the Use of Hypnosis

APA**	1998	*Principles of Medical Ethics With Annotations Especially Applicable to Psychiatry*
APA*	1994	Guidelines for Child Custody Evaluations in Divorce Proceedings
	1999	Test Security: Protecting the Integrity of Tests
	2002	Ethical Principles of Psychologists and Code of Conduct
ASPPB	2005	*ASPPB Code of Conduct*
CEGFP	1991	Specialty Guidelines for Forensic Psychologists
CPA	2000	*Canadian Code of Ethics for Psychologists* (3rd ed.)
	2001	*Practice Guidelines for Providers of Psychological Services*
CPPS	1999	Guidelines for Psychological Evaluations in Child Protection Matters
NAN	2000a	Presence of Third Party Observers During Neuropsychological Testing: Official Statement of the National Academy of Neuropsychology
	2000b	Test Security: Official Position Statement of the National Academy of Neuropsychology
	2000c	The Use of Neuropsychology Test Technicians in Clinical Practice: Official Statement of the National Academy of Neuropsychology
	2003	*Informed Consent: Official Statement of the National Academy of Neuropsychology*[a]
	2003	*Test Security: An Update. Official Statement of the National Academy of Neuropsychology*
	2005	*Independent and Court-Ordered Forensic Neuropsychological Examinations: Official Statement of the National Academy of Neuropsychology*[b]
	2005	Symptom Validity Assessment: Practice Issues and Medical Necessity. NAN Position Paper[c]

Note. AACAP = American Academy of Child and Adolescent Psychiatry; AACN = American Academy of Clinical Neuropsychology; AAP = American Academy of Pediatrics; AAPL = American Academy of Psychiatry and the Law; AERA = American Educational Research Association; AFCC = Association of Family and Conciliation Courts; AMA = American Medical Association; APA** = American Psychiatric Association; APA* = American Psychological Association; ASPPB = Association of State and Provincial Psychology Boards; CEGFP = Committee on Ethical Guidelines for Forensic Psychologists of the American Psychology–Law Society (Division 41) of the American Psychological Association; CPA = Canadian Psychological Association; CPPS = Committee on Professional Practice and Standards; NAN = National Academy of Neuropsychology; NCME = National Council on Measurement in Education. Complete references are available in the reference section.
[a] Johnson-Greene is the lead author.
[b] Bush is the lead author.
[c] Bush et al. are the authors.

DHHS], 1996) took effect in April 2003 and has been a source of confusion for forensic psychologists. This legislation was intended to simplify and protect the confidentiality of electronic billing and transmission of health information and to provide increased patient access to their medical records, including patients' right to amend their medical records to clarify errors. Although those goals may seem logical and straightforward, the legislation evolved into a complex series of administrative rules, with exceptions for certain settings.

Of particular relevance to this chapter is the determination of whether HIPAA applies to forensic services, and if so, to what extent. HIPAA states that information compiled in anticipation of use in civil, criminal, and administrative proceedings is not subject to the same right of review and amendment as is health care information in general (U.S. DHHS, 1996, §164.524(a)(1)(ii)).

Connell and Koocher (2003) opined that forensic practice may not be subject to HIPAA, because (a) forensic services are designed to serve a legal purpose, rather than a therapeutic purpose; (b) forensic services are provided at the request of a party or entity outside the health care system; (c) forensic services fall outside health insurance coverage, because they do not constitute health care; and (d) forensic psychologists do not ordinarily transmit data electronically except in the specific ways for which consent has historically been obtained from the litigant, and (e) no new protections or rights accrue to examinees by way of HIPAA compliance (i.e., no new right of access and amendment of information gathered in anticipation of litigation; U.S. DHHS, 1996, §164.524(a)(1)(ii)).

Legitimate arguments, also noted by Connell and Koocher (2003), posit that forensic practitioners indeed need to become HIPAA compliant. Such arguments include (a) the observation that assessment and diagnosis with respect to an individual's mental condition or functional status may in fact constitute health care, according to HIPAA; as a result, psychologists who provide forensic assessment services may be considered by HIPAA to be covered entities; (b) to obtain health care information about a litigant from other service providers, forensic psychologists must provide assurance that that the information will be handled in a secure way; and (c) the question of whether forensic psychologists are covered entities will likely fall to case law for resolution, and it may prove less expensive and burdensome to become compliant than to become the case that decides the issue.

When considering the applicability of overlapping state and federal laws, the more stringent of the two applies. With regard to HIPAA, this means that the law that provides the most protection of private health care information applies.

Conflicts Between Ethics and Law

Jurisdictional laws provide guidelines for professional behavior that ultimately must be followed. However, psychologists also have a duty to pursue the highest standard of conduct, which may require attempts to compromise with legal authorities when the APA Ethics Code requires a higher standard of professional behavior than does the law. The Introduction and Applicability section of the Ethics Code states,

> If this Ethics Code establishes a higher standard of conduct than is required by law, psychologists must meet the higher ethical standard. If psychologists' ethical responsibilities conflict with law, regulations, or other governing legal authority, psychologists [must] make known their commitment to this Ethics Code and take steps to resolve the conflict in a responsible manner. If the conflict is unresolvable via such means, psychologists may adhere to the requirements of the law, regulations, or other governing authority in keeping with basic principles of human rights.

In many instances, efforts to compromise will result both in the legal system receiving the information or action it requires and in the preservation of the integrity of psychological information or techniques. Although all such attempts will not meet with equal success, the attempts themselves help to educate others about the ethical concerns of psychologists and demonstrate the psychologist's commitment to high practice standards.

A PROPOSED MODEL OF ETHICAL DECISION MAKING IN FORENSIC PSYCHOLOGY

Determining a course of professional behavior that not only avoids ethical misconduct according to an ethics code but also adheres to high aspirational principles requires a commitment to ethical ideals. Determining such a course of action requires access to the necessary tools, and it requires effort and time. Some practitioners may find adherence to the letter of enforceable ethical standards to be sufficient. In our view, however, it is difficult to justify choosing not to pursue the highest standard of ethical behavior available to psychologists. As Knapp and VandeCreek (2003) stated, "Ethics Codes of professions are, by their very nature, incomplete moral codes" (p. 7). Positive ethics requires a shift from an emphasis on misconduct and disciplinary action to an emphasis on the pursuit of one's highest ethical potential (Handelsman, Knapp, & Gottlieb, 2002). The forensic psychologist must understand not simply that certain practices are unethical but, rather, why they are unethical (Shuman & Greenberg, 1998).

Ethical-decision-making models for psychologists have previously been provided (e.g., Canadian Psychological Association, 1991; Haas & Malouf, 2002; Kitchener, 2000; Koocher & Keith-Spiegel, 1998). Knapp and VandeCreek (2003) reviewed these models and identified five common steps: (a) identification of the problem, (b) development of alternatives, (c) evaluation of alternatives, (d) implementation of the best option, and (e) evaluation of the results. Knapp and VandeCreek also noted that these models, although valuable, do not adequately consider emotional and situational factors or the need, in some situations, for an immediate response. They proposed that when considering emotional and situational factors, psychologists engage in self-care activities, become aware of when their own emotional needs begin to interfere with sound professional judgment, and be alert to situational pressures. To best address the need for urgent ethical decision making, they recommended that psychologists anticipate the types of problems that may be encountered in one's practice and then develop decision-making steps for such problems that can be implemented when needed.

The eight-step model proposed in this text incorporates the five common steps of the models reviewed by Knapp and VandeCreek (2003) and integrates the decision-making components that were found to be lacking in those models. This model was designed to provide forensic psychologists with a means to resolve ethical challenges. Given the complexity of many ethical challenges and the range of information and consultation that may be needed to determine an appropriate course of action, it may be beneficial, as Knapp and VandeCreek suggested, for practitioners to anticipate potential ethical conflicts and determine a priori optimal courses of action. The steps of the forensic psychology ethical-decision-making model are as follows: (a) identify the problem, (b) consider the significance of the context and setting, (c) identify and use ethical and legal resources, (d) consider personal beliefs and values, (e) develop possible solutions to the problem, (f) consider the potential consequences of various solutions, (g) choose and implement a course of action, and (h) assess the outcome and implement changes as needed.

Identify the Problem

Some professional activities considered by, or requested of, forensic psychologists are clearly appropriate and ethical, and some are clearly not. However, many options considered by practitioners are ambiguous or present complex layers to be considered. Forensic psychologists must keep in mind that a wide range of potential behaviors may be appropriate when considering courses of action and when reviewing the work of colleagues. A distinction may need to be made between ethical, legal, moral, and professional perspectives. These overlapping concepts may need to be parsed out to clarify the ethical problem or dilemma.

Clearly ethical or unethical behaviors need little explanation or discussion. If one engages in blatantly unethical behavior, one risks a host of negative consequences. If one observes such behavior in a colleague, a course of action must be taken to remedy the situation. However, in the less clear circumstances often encountered in practice, a psychologist may encounter a request or a situation that arouses feelings of uneasiness, a sense that something may be wrong with the situation. In such situations, the psychologist must consider possible reasons for the unease and attempt to narrow down the possibilities, eventually focusing on those elements of the situation that are contributing to the initial feelings of discomfort. For example, a psychologist treating a patient who sustained posttraumatic stress in a motor vehicle accident may be called by the patient's attorney with a request for a report that describes the patient's symptoms, degree of disability, and link between the accident and the posttraumatic stress. The psychologist may be conflicted about the appropriateness of writing such a report. A request such as this that may seem straightforward on the surface may involve a host of issues that would need to be considered by the psychologist. The psychologist would benefit from determining, as specifically as possible, what it is about the situation that is troubling. If such a situation had been considered in advance, the psychologist would likely know exactly how to respond to the request.

Consider the Significance of the Context and Setting

Forensic psychologists work in widely varying settings and contexts. Professional activities that are appropriate in one forensic setting or context may be inappropriate in others. Consequently, some professional guidelines that are relevant in one setting or context may be less relevant or wholly inapplicable in other situations. For example, a forensic psychologist's fee structure may differ, quite appropriately, depending on the nature of the services provided. To the extent that the fee structure may compromise objectivity, the distinction made regarding context is of ethical importance.

In any forensic role there may be a number of individuals or institutions to whom or to which obligations are owed. Although this will differ by context, some possible parties to whom obligations may be owed include the following: referral source, client, examinee, patient, guardians of examinee or patient, employing institution, profession of psychology, trier of fact, court, legal system, and society at large. In some contexts, these parties may overlap, whereas in others they are distinct.

Just as there exists a range of individuals or institutions owed obligations, there is a range of obligations that may be owed. In general terms, the forensic psychologist has an obligation to provide competent services that advance the welfare of the individuals and institutions to which obligations are owed, without bringing unjust harm to the other individuals and institutions involved. The nature of the harm to be avoided has been specified as unjust harm. This clarification is provided because, given the adversarial nature of the legal system, many of the opinions offered or determinations made by psychologists may be considered unfavorable and thus harmful to one of the parties involved in a case. Such opinions or determinations are only unethical if they were reached in an inappropriate manner.

Identify and Use Ethical and Legal Resources

This step may be the most challenging in the ethical-decision-making process. There exist a number of published resources, sometimes offering conflicting guidance, relevant to ethical issues encountered in forensic psychology. Nevertheless, by using both the published and interpersonal resources described in this section, the forensic psychologist can likely find solid footing when determining courses of action that are consistent with ethical practice.

The various resources are presented here in an order consistent with a deductive or top-down method of ethical reasoning and decision making (Beauchamp & Childress, 2001). This method involves applying a general rule to a specific case. First, assess the foundational values. General bioethical principles, the ethics codes of professional organizations, and jurisdictional laws all reflect the values of a society. Examples of North American values include the right to self-determination and the right to adequate health care. These values underlie general bioethical principles, such as respect for a client's autonomy and the need to "do no harm" to the parties served by the health care professional. Determining the values underlying a given ethical standard or law will help to clarify the spirit behind the letter of the standard or law and, by extension, will help to clarify the appropriate course action (Behnke et al., 2003). Behnke et al. (2003) advised that an ethical dilemma be approached by first asking the following questions: "What values are at issue? And how can I act consistent with those values?" (p. 225).

Second, determine the applicable bioethical principles. Beauchamp and Childress (2001) presented a model of bioethical principles reflecting society's fundamental values. Their model, which has been widely adopted across health care disciplines, posits four core principles: autonomy, beneficence, nonmaleficence, and justice. As previously indicated in the chapter, these principles are clearly evident in the 2002 APA Ethics Code.

Applying the Beauchamp and Childress (2001) model to ethical challenges in forensic psychology can be of considerable value in determining an appropriate course of action. However, dilemmas emerge or increase in complexity in situations in which one value is pitted against another. For example, from an ethical perspective, releasing raw test data to a patient may, depending on the context, be consistent with respecting the patient's autonomy, but it may also result in psychological harm to the patient and harm to society at large depending on the uses to which the data are put. Weighing the relative importance of the principles involved and attempting to strike a balance that satisfies the greater good is the task of the forensic psychologist. Of course, such determinations need not, and often should not, be made in isolation.

Third, review relevant professional ethics codes. Ethics codes are developed to reduce the vagueness inherent in professional values (Beauchamp & Childress, 2001). The APA Ethics Code provides guidance for ethical psychological practice. Whereas the Ethics Code's General Principles are aspirational in nature, the Ethical Standards provide more concrete dicta for ethical practice and should be consulted to achieve an ethical solution. The Ethical Standards are the enforceable minimum level of ethical conduct for psychologists who are APA members or whose state boards have adopted the Ethics Code as the professional regulations or rules of practice for licensed psychologists.

Fourth, psychologists must be familiar with the jurisdictional laws that regulate the profession of psychology where they practice. State and federal laws offer specific guidance on how to manage fundamental aspects of psychological practice; however, more specific practices pertaining to psychological specialty areas may not be adequately addressed by statutory or case law.

Fifth, refer to position statements (i.e., *white papers*) of relevant professional psychological associations. These position statements offer clarification of details of practice areas that are beyond the scope of an ethics code. Many of these statements are readily available from the Web sites of the organizations authoring or endorsing them. The SGFP, currently under revision, provide ethical guidance specific to forensic activities (Committee on Ethical Guidelines for Forensic Psychologists, 1991).

Sixth, review journal articles, books, and book chapters: "Theory and principle are only starting points and general guides for the development of norms of appropriate conduct. They are supplemented by paradigm cases of right action, empirical data, organizational experience, and the like" (Beauchamp & Childress, 2001, p. 2). General ethics texts provide coverage of ethical issues of concern to forensic psychologists and may offer vignettes specific to forensic practice. Forensic psychology books cover, to varying degrees, many of the practice issues that are of ethical concern, and some provide specific ethics chapters. In addition, texts from related psychology specialty areas, such as child and family psychology and neuropsychology, include chapters that address forensically relevant ethical issues. Thus, there exist many published resources that can assist the forensic psychologist who is anticipating or experiencing ethical challenges.

Seventh, consult colleagues. Such consultation may occur informally through discussions with colleagues and formally through contact with ethics committees, or both. The experiences of colleagues who have faced similar ethical challenges and the collective knowledge and experience of ethics committees may provide invaluable assistance to the psychologist facing an ethical dilemma. Consultation with others in one's own jurisdiction may offer the advantage of sensitivity to both the legal and ethical aspects of a case. However, one might also need, in certain circumstances, to seek consultation from outside the geographic area to preserve confidentiality of case involvement or of details of the matter. It is useful to establish several collegial consultative relationships and also to seek expertise to address the relevant issues of the matter at hand. The consultation may be formalized, even on a case-by-case basis, by establishing a consultation agreement, retaining the consultant at an hourly fee, and requesting that the consultant maintain a record of the consultation. Such consultation can then be identified, if later needed, as one of the ways the psychologist strived to meet the ethical challenge in a professional and thoughtful way.

Consider Personal Beliefs and Values

In addition to, or at times in contrast to, the collective values of a society that were previously described, the psychologist may endorse a particular value to some degree along a continuum. Forensic psychologists have a responsibility to evaluate the degree to which their personal moral positions are consistent with those of the larger society and the organizations with which they are involved. To the extent possible, they should attempt to understand their biases and the potential impact that their values and biases have on their professional and ethical decision making. Psychologists may also draw on personal values other than those reflected in a model of professional ethics, such as their religion or cultural background. It is critically important that forensic psychologists, whose work often involves matters laden with moral and values implications, attempt to understand the potential influences of their personal beliefs on their professional behavior.

Develop Possible Solutions to the Problem

When one is faced with an ethical dilemma, inaction is typically not an ethical option. The legal counsel that one may obtain may address the issue from a risk-management perspective, arguing for temporary inaction or for avoidance of efforts at resolution that might incur liability, whereas the principles by which the psychologist practices may argue for action that remediates potential suffering on the part of a party in the situation. The complex dilemmas that pit one ethical principle against another, or ethical against legal considerations, may tax the most thoughtful practitioner.

Generating a list of possible solutions requires integration of the significance of the context, information obtained from available resources, and personal beliefs and values. In some situations, the best course of action may be clear upon such consideration. However, in other ethically challenging situations, practitioners may need to generate a number of potential solutions in as much detail as possible. Consider the example of releasing raw test data to an opposing attorney. When provided with an appropriate client release, there are a variety of options that the forensic psychologist should consider. Some of these options include (a) immediately releasing the data as requested, (b) refusing to release the data on the basis of published professional guidelines, (c) offering to release the data to a psychologist retained by the opposing attorney, (d) requesting a court order to release the data, and (e) requesting a protective order from the court.

Consider the Potential Consequences of Various Solutions

Once possible solutions to the ethical problem have been developed, potential consequences must be considered. Both positive and negative consequences must be anticipated. Just as the relative importance of underlying values was assessed, the potential positive and negative consequences of each action may need to be weighed to determine the best course of action. In the example of releasing raw data, a variety of potential consequences emerge. Spending time and resources striving to safeguard the test data, which includes the materials on which responses are recorded, may seem futile in the adversarial forum where rights to discovery of such materials are legally defined. In contrast, the psychologist may believe that it is ethically preferable to minimize the opportunity for nonpsychologists to get access to test questions and stimuli, thus justifying the expenditure of time and resources. However, by taking steps that may be perceived as obstructive or oppositional, the psychologist may fear repercussions such as antagonizing the court or the attorneys, thereby reducing good will with those with whom one wishes to work. Thus, the potential consequences may extend beyond solely ethical considerations to those with business and other implications. Forensic psychologists must consider potential consequences, weigh their options, and pursue the highest ethical option available.

Choose and Implement a Course of Action

Once potential solutions have been examined and consequences considered, the practitioner must select and implement the most appropriate course of action. The timing of the action may be critical to its success. Depending on the issues involved and the context, the course of action may need to occur quickly or may need to be delayed. Again using the example of a request for test data, the request may have attached to it an instruction to delay release for a specified period of time, to provide counsel time to consult with the litigant, if necessary, and to file a motion to quash the request or subpoena. Consultation with colleagues may be particularly valuable in weighing the best time to respond to situations in which timing must be taken into account.

Assess the Outcome and Implement Changes as Needed

With many difficult ethical decisions, the chosen action will likely be unsatisfactory to one or more of the parties involved. The psychologist should be prepared to receive and respond to feedback about the decisions made and actions taken. Similarly, the psychologist must evaluate the effectiveness of his or her own decision or action and implement changes as needed.

APPLYING APPROPRIATE RISK-MANAGEMENT STRATEGIES IN FORENSIC PRACTICE

In 1984, Alan Stone wrote, "The philosophers say life is a moral adventure; I would add that to choose a career in forensic psychiatry is to choose to increase the risks of that moral adventure" (p. 73). Psychologists engaging in forensic professional activities enter an environment with moral, ethical, and professional challenges that are often quite different from those found in clinical practice. These challenges and their associated potential ethical pitfalls put the unprepared psychologist at considerable risk for professional misconduct. A significant contribution to decreasing one's vulnerability to professional misconduct can be made by striving to understand the laws that govern one's practice. As Sales and Miller (1993) indicated, however,

> Most professionals do not know about, much less understand, most of the laws that affect their practice, the services they render, and the clients they serve . . . not knowing about the laws that affect the services they render can result in incompetent performance of, and liability for, the mental health professional. (p. 1)

Continuing education in the areas of one's psychological specialty, the laws that regulate one's practice, the interface of the specialty practice with the legal system, and risk management itself are all necessary for maximally reducing the likelihood of engaging in professional misconduct. However, knowledge is not enough. Forensic psychologists must be committed to applying that knowledge in a manner that is consistent with ethical practice. Where professional competence has been established and is being maintained, the greatest risk to ethical misconduct in forensic psychology seems to be the potential influence of bias. Bennett, Bryant, VandenBos, and Greenwood (1990) stated, "Too often, we fail to evaluate our own performance, attitudes, behaviors, and work skills objectively in terms of the ethics and practice guidelines of the profession" (p. 7). For example, a strong belief in a particular methodology or symptom etiology may overshadow objectivity (Bennett et al., 1990). Bias in this context, however, addresses not just a philosophical preference for one aspect of the professional literature or another but also the intentional modification of behaviors, written opinions, or testimony designed solely to support the position of the retaining party. Bias can exert its influence even when the psychologist is well armed with information about the professionally correct course of action.

To justify one's positions and behaviors, clear and detailed documentation of the rationale should be maintained. As Behnke et al. (2003) stated, "*the process by which a clinician decides what to do* becomes as important as the decision itself" (p. 13). Documentation that the psychologist understood the values at stake and followed a rational process of ethical decision making will, if necessary, inform any outside reviewer that the ethical challenge was addressed in a thoughtful and systematic manner. Such documentation of the decision-making process will be the forensic psychologist's best protection against liability (Behnke et al., 2003).

As G. W. Lynch (1993) stated, "Historically, there has been tension, and indeed antipathy at times, between attorneys and mental health professionals" (p. 7). Nevertheless, when issues of professional liability are in doubt, psychologists would be well served to consult both their own attorney and their professional liability insurance carrier. In considering the consultation, it is essential to keep in mind that the interests of the attorney or insurance carrier may overlap with one's own, but in some respects, may not, and at the end of the day, one must be comfortable that the action to be taken reflects the values and ethics held to be meaningful.

2

THE REFERRAL

The process that ultimately results in the provision of forensic psychological evaluation or treatment services begins when the psychologist is contacted by an interested individual or organization. Initial contacts are often made by the individual or organization that will become the retaining party. The nature of the relationship between the psychologist and the retaining party and the manner in which the relationship is established have ethical implications for the remainder of the psychologist's involvment in the case.

THE RETAINING-PARTY/EXAMINER RELATIONSHIP

The fundamental human value underlying the retaining-party/ examiner relationship is that all parties are entitled to a clear understanding of the expectations of the others involved to make an informed decision about whether to engage in the relationship. The court is entitled to expect from its experts the clarity of purpose on which reliable testimony is based and can best derive benefit from expert testimony borne out of clearly defined roles. The principle of autonomy reflects this informed decision-making process.

When agreeing to accept a case that involves or may involve litigation, psychologists should perform each step of their work in a manner defensible within the legal forum (Hartlage, 2003). The relationship between the retaining party and the examiner is the foundation on which all psychological services are based: "Clarifying issues will tend to ensure that later conflict does not develop about the conduct of the evaluation or testimony" (Melton, Petrila, Poythress, & Slobogin, 1997, p. 82). A lack of clarity among involved parties regarding roles and responsibilities renders the working relationship vulnerable to subsequent misunderstanding and conflict and in itself represents ethical misconduct (Standard 3.07, Third-Party Requests for Services, of the American Psychological Association's [APA's] Ethics Code, 2002).

As Barsky and Gould (2002) noted, "A vital first step in becoming an intentional witness is to identify your roles" (p. 27). Identifying one's role is not always as straightforward as might be anticipated. Clarifying the questions to be answered or forensic issues to be addressed in the context of a matter is essential to understanding one's role. The forensic issues may involve a plaintiff's or criminal defendant's cognitive or psychological functioning or the relationships among individuals. Increasing the decision maker's understanding of such functioning serves the larger legal question on which the case is based, such as the plaintiff's right to compensation, the innocence or guilt of the accused, or the allocation of parental responsibilities in a way that serves the best interests of the child. Therefore, when identifying one's role, "an important first step is to identify the forensic issues contained in the legal questions that have triggered the need for the evaluation" (Heilbrun, 2001, p. 22).

Established through discussions between the psychologist and the retaining party and at least partially deriving from statutory or case law is an understanding about the nature of the information the psychologist gives the examinee and the extent to which information obtained during the evaluation process will be kept confidential or, conversely, will be discoverable (Melton et al., 1997). Thus, the psychologist and the retaining party must be clear about their mutual expectations from the outset: "Clarifications such as these at the early stages of consultation will result in a smoother relationship as the case proceeds" (Melton et al., 1997, p. 83).

Objectivity in the Role of Forensic Expert

When retained as forensic experts, psychologists should anticipate attempts by attorneys or clients to elicit opinions for which adequate support does not exist (Barsky & Gould, 2002). This may occur at trial, when tensions are high and there is little opportunity to re-examine and discuss expectations and resolve conflicting interpretations of the data:

> Despite efforts to achieve objectivity, a good psychologist is highly motivated to help the patient. The expert who agrees to serve as both

treating health care provider and forensic expert is on thin ice ethically because of the potential conflict in these dual roles. (Lees-Haley & Cohen, 1999, p. 445)

By anticipating this possibility at the outset, the psychologist may be better prepared to maintain previously agreed-on boundaries. The success of a patient's litigation should not be the direct concern of the testifying expert. Rather, the expert's carefully developed opinion, and the sound data underlying it, remains the focus. The task is to assist the court by providing reliable information relevant to the matter to be decided.

Psychologists retained as forensic experts should also consider whether they were retained because their opinions tend to be predictable; that is, their opinions consistently reflect advocacy for a particular belief or they consistently favor the retaining party, rather than being based on the facts of a given case. Psychologists are encouraged to assess their practices and take steps to maximize their potential for arriving at impartial conclusions. Such steps include ensuring professional competence (discussed later in this chapter) and engaging in self-examination.

Self-examination should assess past objectivity and maximize current and future objectivity. To assess past objectivity, practitioners may calculate an objectivity quotient, determined by dividing the number of cases in which there was agreement with the referring attorney by the total number of cases (Brodsky, 1991). Agreement with referring parties in greater than 80% of cases is considered consistent with excessive favorability and preexisting bias. This formulation is to be contrasted with the illogical concept focusing on percent of opinions that favor one side or the other in forensic proceedings (e.g., 50% prosecution and 50% defense, or whatever percentage plaintiff vs. defense). Although Brodsky's formulation reasonably addresses the concern of bias, the second concept may actually reflect bias when the expert changes an opinion to favor the retaining side. Take, for example, the clinical researcher whose published research demonstrates repressed memories are false. The examiner will rarely be called as an expert by the side of a plaintiff alleging childhood sexual abuse on the basis of repressed memory evidence; if this were to occur, and the expert disregarded or "explained away" the research to support the plaintiff's claim, one might suspect bias in favor of retaining parties.

Self-examination questions, such as those offered by Sweet and Moulthrop (1999b), offer practitioners a possible means of maximizing current and future objectivity. Such debiasing procedures have been criticized for their lack of empirical support (see, e.g., Lees-Haley, 1999; response by Sweet & Moulthrop, 1999a). However, given the current absence of empirically supported debiasing procedures, psychologists practicing in forensic contexts will be well served by ensuring professional competence (e.g., through appropriate education, training, experience, and peer review of one's work) and using self-examination techniques.

Advocacy in the Role of Trial Consultant

In assuming the role of trial consultant, the psychologist enters a relationship with an attorney that is different from that of an attorney and a testifying expert, in that advocacy may more reasonably be expected in the former. Nevertheless, the nature of the psychologist's role requires clarification at the outset. In this context, the psychologist essentially joins the retaining attorney's team to bring psychological expertise to the partisan adversarial process. Impartiality is not required of the trial consultant, but the psychologist trial consultant who holds a place on the "trial team" is cautioned against agreeing to transition into or concurrently participate in the case as an examining or testifying expert (Brodsky, 1999). Although some authors have maintained that a consultant can assume a partisan role in assisting an attorney's case and serve as an impartial evaluator until the time of trial, at which point only the role of impartial evaluator is maintained (e.g., Halleck, 1980), separating the acceptable bias of the consultant from the necessary objectivity of the evaluator is an extremely difficult endeavor to undertake, if possible at all. Heilbrun (2001) identified as an emerging principle the "single-role" maxim that should be familiar to the practicing forensic psychologist and advised declining a referral when impartiality would likely be jeopardized.

Not uncommonly, psychologists may find this distinction between testifying expert and consultant difficult to maintain. For example, an attorney may ask a psychologist that she has retained as a testifying expert for feedback regarding the opposing expert's report and invoke discussion about a point of disagreement between the experts. The testifying expert, in explaining the source of the difference, essentially offers the attorney a roadmap for cross-examining the opposing expert. Although there is no clear line distinguishing the appropriate contribution of a testifying expert from that of a nontestifying, consulting expert, practitioners may help clarify the appropriate course of action by examining their motivations. Being motivated to clarify genuine professional disagreement and its genesis, to assist an attorney in making appropriate use of one's opinion, the testifying expert is on solid ground. When the motivation is to contribute as a member of the trial team, sharing its goal to win the case, the psychologist has become an advocate whose opinions should not be offered as objective expertise.

COMPETENCE

Psychological services, to be effective and useful to consumers, must be performed competently. Such professional competence is typically obtained through a combination of education, formal practical training, and experience (Melton et al., 1997). Competence is not universal; that is, competence in one area of psychology does not imply competence in another area. This is true across and within specialty areas of practice. Within specialty areas, competence does not necessarily transfer across patient populations or clinical settings. This specificity of competence is particularly significant in forensic settings or contexts, in which specialized knowledge of the rules or laws governing the activity is essential. Further, competence in a particular psychology specialty area does not necessarily translate into competence in performing that specialty in a forensic context or setting (Heilbrun, 2001; Nagy, 2000). Psychologists who provide expert testimony without having had proper specialty training, including training specific to forensic practice, are practicing beyond the scope of their competence (Slick & Iverson, 2003).

The concept of professional competence is based on the fundamental human value that people have the right to psychological services that are not harmful and that provide the assistance that they purport to provide. The bioethical principles of nonmaleficence and beneficence reflect this underlying value. Psychologists who lack the necessary competence to provide their services in forensic contexts may not be able to provide an acceptable level of accuracy and reliability, and risk harming those with whom they interact professionally.

The 2002 APA Ethics Code requires professional competence (Standards 2.01, Boundaries of Competence, and 2.04, Bases for Scientific and Professional Judgments) but allows an exception for services provided in emergency situations when services would otherwise be unavailable (Standard 2.02, Providing Services in Emergencies). When provided in this context, services are discontinued when the emergency has ended or more appropriate services are available. The Specialty Guidelines for Forensic Psychologists (SGFP; Committee on Ethical Guidelines for Forensic Psychologists, 1991) stipulate that the SGFP, including those related to professional competence, apply to psychologists who regularly engage in forensic activities. Thus, psychologists whose professional activities regularly involve interaction with the legal system are responsible for demonstrating competence to perform their activities in that context.

Just as competence is not universal, it is not static (Standard 2.03, Maintaining Competence). Competence must be maintained through continuing education and relevant professional activities (Blau, 1998). However, difficulty may lie in determining what represents competence in forensic psychology. Psychologists who engage in forensic activities represent a range of specializations. Such diversity is important for assisting the court with the range of questions that emerge; however, ambiguity regarding qualifications may emerge in individual cases. In fact, despite the existence of a division of the APA devoted to psychological and legal issues (i.e., Division 41 [American Psychology–Law Society]) and the creation of the American Board of Forensic Psychology, there remains debate within the field regarding the definition of *forensic psychology* (Brigham, 1999; Heilbrun, 2001). In the individual case, however, this difficulty is reduced somewhat in that it is the court that determines who qualifies as an expert for the matter at hand. Rule 702 of the *Federal Rules of Evidence for the United States Courts and Magistrates* (FRE; 1975) and state laws define who is qualified to testify as an expert. The psychologist is responsible for accurate representation of the knowledge, skill, experience, training, and education that compose the relevant credentials (Standard 5.01a, Avoidance of False or Deceptive Statements; Barsky & Gould, 2002; FRE 702). The court then weighs the probable relevance and reliability of the testimony to be offered in determining whether to qualify the proffered witness as an expert whose opinion testimony will assist the trier of fact (FRE 702). Nevertheless, that psychologists must only provide services within their areas of competence is considered an established principle (Heilbrun, 2001).

FINANCIAL ARRANGEMENTS

The strength of the judicial system derives from society's expectation that the decisions rendered by the court are just. To that end, society anticipates that expert witnesses involved in serving the court will perform their duties objectively. Practices that have the potential to negatively affect objectivity, and by extension justice, must be carefully considered by psychologists. The manner in which the psychologist's fees are arranged is one factor that has the potential to significantly interfere with, or appear to interfere with, objectivity. When a psychologist's fees are contingent on the outcome of a legal case, the psychologist is vulnerable to intentionally or unintentionally producing a report or testimony that favors the retaining party. As a result, the SGFP state as follows:

> Forensic psychologists do not provide professional services to parties to a legal proceeding on the basis of "contingent fees," when those services involve the offering of expert testimony to a court or administrative body, or when they call upon the psychologist to make affirmations or

representations intended to be relied upon by third parties. (SGFP IV, B, Relationships)

It can be argued that contingency fees pose no greater threat to objectivity than does retention by any party with a stake in the outcome of an adversarial proceeding. Although some attorneys appreciate an objective expert opinion even when it does not support their position—and attorneys may articulate just that position—the expert is well aware that sometimes attorneys are seeking an opinion that does support their case. If the psychologist's opinion does not support the retaining attorney's case, the attorney may attempt to massage the opinion into shape. The psychologist who holds firm to the data is sharply aware that the attorney may be lost as a referral source. Thus, it could be argued that psychologists who are retained by one side in a legal case, regardless of how they choose to bill for their services, are subject to the same threats to objectivity. Although it is true that the potential for biased reporting exists for all forensic experts, those whose fees are directly related to litigation outcome face a greater threat to objectivity and a clearer appearance of compromised objectivity. The provision of an opinion for which payment is contingent on the outcome of the case is both unethical and strongly discouraged in the professional literature (Heilbrun, 2001). Thus, contingency fees should not be accepted (American Academy of Psychiatry and the Law, 1995; Committee on Ethical Guidelines for Forensic Psychologists, 1991) except when one is working as a nontestifying expert in trial consultation.

The nature of trial consultation, in which a psychologist is retained by an attorney to assist in preparing the case against the other side, raises an exception to the proscription against contingency fees. In this role, the psychologist, like the retaining attorney, assumes a position for one party. The role is not to inform the trier of fact. Given that the objective review and presentation of information to the retaining attorney is expected to clarify the mental health issues in a way that will assist the attorney in case presentation and therefore strengthen the attorney's case, the role is not one of neutrality (Heilbrun, 2001). In this context, the manner in which the psychologist is paid does not alter the service provided. Because impartiality is not a requirement of the consultant role, it cannot be affected by contingency fees. Thus, it would be ethical for the nontestifying consulting psychologist, like the attorney, to choose to accept payment for services contingent on the outcome of the case.

Another potential financial arrangement that may provide the psychologist with incentive to deviate from ethical practice is charging higher fees for testimony (Heilbrun, 2001). Although the added stress and inconvenience that can be associated with testimony may seem to justify increased payment, the availability of higher fees may provide motivation to engage in inappropriate activities to increase the likelihood that one may be asked to testify. One such example would be omitting an important piece of information from a report and then informing the attorney of the omission and the need to elicit the information during testimony. The psychologist wishing to avoid the appearance of ethically questionable practice is advised to avoid charging higher fees for testimony.

Ethically preferable financial arrangements include setting fixed rates for a given service, which may be required in some states, and when billing an hourly rate, doing so in a manner that is consistent across various forensic services provided. In considering billing options, the goal is not only to be adequately and fairly compensated for one's services but also to limit the potential to have one's opinions or work product swayed by the possibility of increased revenue. Psychologists and their clients should establish compensation and billing arrangements as early as possible in the professional relationship (Standard 6.04, Fees and Financial Arrangements).

CASE 1: HANDLING REFERRALS IN PERSONAL INJURY LITIGATION

A personal injury attorney contacts a psychologist who has experience working with people who have been involved in car accidents. The attorney explains that her 63-year-old client was involved in a motor vehicle accident a month ago and, in her opinion, has posttraumatic stress disorder (PTSD). She is making the referral for psychological treatment because her client lives alone, has no close relatives, and does not know how to access the services he needs. The attorney explains that the patient's no-fault car insurance will be the payment source. She offers to fax the police report and ambulance and emergency room records, and she requests an appointment for her client. The psychologist, feeling a little uncomfortable about the proposed fee arrangement, nevertheless accepts the referral and provides an appointment time for the litigant to be seen. After hanging up, the psychologist reflects on the nature of the referral.

Analysis

Identify the Problem

The psychologist accepted a referral from an attorney without exploring his possible role in the litigation. The psychologist asked no questions about the attorney's expectations and conveyed no information regarding his practices with respect to patients who are involved in litigation.

Consider the Significance of the Context and Setting

This apparent clinical referral occurred within the context of civil litigation. The attorney, although possibly interested in the psychological welfare of her client, likely had additional motivation for initiating psychological treatment. The attorney seemed to have made the diagnosis of PTSD and was sending records that the psychologist had not requested and may or may not have found necessary. The psychologist, in musing about this referral, considered that the attorney would likely be making requests of him once his initial assessment was performed and treatment was underway. He wondered whether he should have addressed these expectations proactively, before accepting the referral.

Identify and Use Ethical and Legal Resources

A fundamental societal value is the right of its members, whether involved in litigation or not, to access appropriate psychological services. An additional value is that society at large, through increases in insurance premiums, should not be expected to pay for health care services that are undertaken to strengthen one's lawsuit. These values are consistent with bioethical principles: beneficence, nonmaleficence, and justice. The psychologist has a responsibility to assist an appropriate patient (beneficence). At the same time, he also must avoid harming the patient (nonmaleficence), which may occur through entering into multiple, potentially conflicting, roles without thoroughly clarifying expectations with the referring attorney and the examinee or treatment recipient (General Principle A; Standards 3.05, Multiple Relationships; 3.07, Third-Party Requests for Services; and 3.10, Informed Consent). The psychologist has ethical and legal obligations to bill the appropriate party for services provided (General Principles C, Integrity, and D, Justice; Standards 6.04a, Fees and Financial Arrangements, and 6.04b). If the symptoms experienced by the patient predate or are otherwise not related to the accident, it would be illegal to bill the no-fault carrier. The psychologist had a responsibility to discuss with the attorney during the initial consultation any factors that may affect the attorney's decision to use the psychologist's services or the psychologist's decision to accept the referral (SGFP IV, A and D2, Relationships).

The blurring of roles is one of the most frequent reasons for ethics complaints against psychologists in custody cases (Heilbrun, 2001). In addition to role-clarity problems in forensic matters, maintaining multiple roles can have a negative effect in a therapeutic relationship. When a clinician is asked to monitor a patient and report the findings to an outside authority, for example, the clinician may have difficulty maintaining the trust of the patient (Barsky & Gould, 2002) and the patient may be less than forthcoming with the therapist. In forensic contexts, role clarification is critically important for all parties, particularly because the assumptions generally held about psychological treatment, such as the confidential and helping nature of the relationship, generally do not apply. Professional guidelines, then, are clear on the dangers of assuming multiple roles. State psychological guidelines also generally echo the standards and guidelines on this issue.

In the present case, once the referral was accepted, the relevant issues of potential role conflict would need to be discussed not only with the referring attorney but also with the patient (litigant; SGFP V, B, Confidentiality and Privilege). However, no laws of that state were found that applied to clarification of roles.

Consider Personal Beliefs and Values

This psychologist believes that any individual reporting symptoms that seem to be consistent with PTSD deserves access to his services. He is generally not concerned about where the referral comes from; however, the nature of this referral was somewhat different for him in that the attorney seemed to have proposed a diagnosis and was sending records that the psychologist typically did not request. Because he had not been retained by the attorney, he preferred to be open to, and accepting of, the patient's experiences. Based on his understanding, if the patient reported that the symptoms emerged or worsened following the automobile accident, then the no-fault carrier would be the appropriate payor.

Develop Possible Solutions to the Problem

The psychologist, feeling somewhat uneasy about the referral, considered four options. First, he considered refusing the referral and possibly suggesting alternative treatment providers. Second, he considered accepting the referral and not worrying about any unexplored expectations at this time. Third, he considered calling the attorney back to obtain further clarification about the attorney's expectations of the nature of his involvement in the matter. Fourth, he considered contacting a colleague to get a second opinion.

Consider the Potential Consequences of Various Solutions

The psychologist considered possible beneficial and adverse effects associated with each of the possible solutions that he had identified. First, he believed that declining the referral and suggesting alternative clinicians without further clarifying expectations would have no significant impact on the patient either way but may not be good for his practice from a business perspective. Second, the psychologist thought that accepting the referral without clarifying expectations could be harmful for all parties at some point during the course of treatment. He was most concerned about the potential harm to his relationship with the patient and, thus, the patient's psychological state should different expectations about the psychologist's role in the litigation emerge during the course of treatment. Additionally, although he would not be accepting the patient into treatment for purpose of assisting the patient's legal case, the psychologist also did not want to interfere with the legal case and the ability of the patient to receive compensation for damages resulting from the accident. Furthermore, the psychologist did not want to unnecessarily hurt the case for the attorney. The psychologist believed that each of these potential adverse consequences, in addition to harming others, had the potential to negatively affect his reputation and professional standing in the community. Third, the psychologist believed that contacting the attorney for clarification would help to clarify expectation so that all parties were in agreement from the outset; however, the thought that such a call may be perceived as offensive by some attorneys may result in the current patient and future patients being referred to another clinician. Fourth, the psychologist believed that seeking a colleague's advice could only be of value.

Choose and Implement a Course of Action

The psychologist did not believe that declining the referral or referring to someone else was necessary. He believed that he could work out the potential conflicts and still provide the patient with appropriate treatment. However, having reflected on the relevant values and ethical guidelines, he believed that the attorney's expectations should be addressed in some way before treating the patient. He thought that a reasonable option would be to call the attorney to clarify expectations, but he also thought that it might be more appropriate to discuss expectations with the patient, without further involving the attorney. However, he wanted to know what others would do, so he chose to call an experienced colleague.

Assess the Outcome and Implement Changes as Needed

The colleague suggested that the most ethically appropriate course of action would be to call the referring attorney prior to seeing the patient to clarify expectations. Indeed, when the psychologist called, the attorney clarified that although the patient's mental health was the first priority, she would be asking for periodic reports on the patient's accident-related psychiatric disability and treatment. The psychologist responded that he appreciated the referral but that he could not promise such reports, as he had not yet met with the patient and had no idea about the patient's psychiatric status or his interest in having that information shared with anyone. The attorney, seemingly losing patience, indicated that she had a number of such clients and was looking for someone to whom she could refer them, hoping that it could be this psychologist, but only if he were "sensitive to litigation issues." The psychologist stated that he would be glad to have the additional referrals, but he maintained his position—an unwillingness to commit prematurely to periodic reports. The attorney said she would send her client somewhere else, and hung up. The psychologist, frustrated by the attorney's determination to select a clinician on the basis of the clinician's willingness to endorse her position, was satisfied that he had made the right decision.

3

COLLECTION AND REVIEW
OF INFORMATION

One of the cardinal differences between most forensic and clinical evaluations is the nature and extent of the background information that is sought and reviewed prior to the rendering of an opinion or the provision of a report (Heilbrun, Warren, & Picarello, 2003). A thorough review of background information allows the forensic psychologist to support opinions with a degree of confidence that may not be attainable in some clinical contexts. The fundamental values relevant to the collection and review of background information are the examinee's right to privacy and the judicial system's right to have expert opinion derived from all information relevant to the formulation of that opinion. These values translate into the ethical principles of autonomy and justice. The potential for conflict between these two values is lessened in many forensic evaluation contexts because the examinee who has raised his or her mental functioning as a legal issue has waived the right to privacy with regard to background information that may be relevant to prior mental functioning.[1]

---

[1] This is not true, of course, when the court develops a concern regarding the mental health of a defendant and raises, *sua sponte*, a request for evaluation or when, in family law matters, the court seeks information regarding the mental health of a party whose capacity to parent has been challenged, or a child has alleged abuse and the court orders an evaluation of the child. Occasions arise, then, when the forensic practitioner must be concerned about the potential intrusion into or violation of a vulnerable party's rights and society's interest in autonomy, beneficence, and justice, to avoid malfeasance.

BASES FOR OPINIONS

Psychologists "base the opinions contained in their recommendations, reports, and diagnostic or evaluative statements, including forensic testimony, on information and techniques sufficient to substantiate their findings" (Standard 9.01a, Bases for Assessments, of the American Psychological Association's [APA's] Ethics Code, 2002) and document in their reports the sources of information on which their conclusions rest (Standard 6.01, Documentation of Professional and Scientific Work and Maintenance of Records). In addition, in forensic contexts, psychologists examine the issue from perspectives that differ from those of the referring party, and they consider and rule out plausible rival hypotheses when making determinations (Specialty Guidelines for Forensic Psychologists [SGFP; Committee on Ethical Guidelines for Forensic Psychologists, 1991] VI, C, Methods and Procedures).

The background information obtained "should be guided by relevance to the forensic issues and validity of the different sources" (Heilbrun, 2001, p. 107). The use of a multisource, multimethod assessment strategy to gather and review reliable and relevant information is a valuable approach to competent forensic assessment (Denney & Wynkoop, 2000; Heilbrun, 2001; Heilbrun et al., 2003; McLearen, Pietz, & Denney, 2004). Forensic evaluation generally includes the use of measures or indicators to illuminate the examinee's response style and response validity. As Rogers (1997) noted, "in spite of variability across settings, the combined prevalence of inconsistent, malingered, and defensive response styles is much too large to ignore, even under the best circumstances" (p. 5).

The sources of information should provide incremental validity; that is, each piece of information, if it is relevant, should contribute to form a full and accurate understanding of the examinee. Inaccurate information or information that is obtained from a source that lacks credibility, if given much weight, lessens the accuracy of the evaluation findings. The use of multiple sources of information helps to provide (a) independent corroboration of essential aspects of the examinee's history; (b) essential information about past mental states that may be relevant to forensic questions; and (c) observational data from a variety of contexts, thus increasing the likelihood that they are representative.

The *Daubert v. Merrell Dow Pharmaceuticals* (1993) decision, like Rule 702 of the *Federal Rules of Evidence for the United States Courts and Magistrates* (1975), emphasized relevance and reliability of evidence as the most important criteria for acceptance of scientific evidence in federal court. Information that is considered legally relevant is that which directly relates to the psycholegal issue, such as a criminal defendant's mental state at the time of an offense, an individual's capacity to create a will, or the capacity of a suspect to voluntarily confess to a crime.

Review of Records

The collection and review of relevant records is an essential aspect of a thorough forensic evaluation (Grisso, 2003; Heilbrun, 2001). For example, documentation of a plaintiff's preaccident level of functioning, as found in school, work, or military records, is needed to establish a baseline against which postaccident behavior can be compared (McLearen et al., 2004). Records pertaining to postaccident injury and functioning, such as medical records, are necessary for establishing injury severity and subsequent signs and symptoms of impairment and disability.

Comparison of preaccident and postaccident records is used to determine whether functioning at the time of the evaluation represents a change. As part of a multisource, multimethod assessment strategy, such data can be used to confirm or disconfirm the plaintiff's self-report. However, the medical records of other professionals provide opportunity for prior invalid symptom reporting to affect one's own professional judgment (Bieliauskas, 1999). For example, neurological reports at times conclude with diagnoses of neurological disorders based on patient self-report, despite normal examination findings. Similarly, the parent who is attempting to gain an upper hand in a contested custody matter may cause to be created both psychotherapeutic and medical records documenting alleged symptoms of abuse or neglect of the child by falsely reporting symptoms or events. The unsuspecting nonforensic health services professional is less likely to maintain suspended judgment and seek corroboration and more likely, in the interest of risk management or out of naivete, to document a diagnostic impression based on report alone. In addition, reports of negative psychiatric histories may be misleading. Potentially inaccurate diagnoses or history, accepted as fact and incorporated into reports, are then perpetuated by other professionals.

Third-Party Information

The use of corroborative data from collateral sources increases both the reliability of the background information obtained and the face validity of the data (Grisso, 2003; Heilbrun, 2001; Heilbrun, Warren, & Picarello 2003; Melton, Petrila, Poythress, & Slobogin, 1997). Information from individuals in a position to observe or interact with the examinee may provide important information to help confirm or refute information obtained through self-report. As stated in the SGFP, "Forensic psychologists attempt to corroborate critical data that form the basis for their professional product" (VI, F1, Methods and Procedures). The nature of the examinee's current abilities and symptoms, and their stability or change over time, is critically significant. Information from third parties may be obtained from unstructured or structured interviews or standardized questionnaires.

Just as examinee self-report may be subject to distortion, the information provided by collateral sources may not be accurate. Inaccurate information may be provided by collateral sources because of bias, a lack of expertise regarding the behaviors in question, suggestibility, and memory loss (Heilbrun, 2001). Examiners can proactively reduce the potential for inaccuracy through the manner in which interview procedures and questions are selected and designed (e.g., see Heilbrun, 2001, pp. 174–175, for specific examples). History obtained from third parties should be verified by multiple sources to the extent possible.

OBTAINING INFORMATION

The timing of the collection of background information may vary depending on the context of the evaluation. At times, records may be obtained prior to meeting with the examinee. In such instances, the content of the records may help to determine the nature of the evaluation that is to be performed. In other cases, it is through the initial meeting with the examinee that a determination is made regarding the specific background information that will be of value, and the examinee's consent to obtain the information may be required.

The psychologist may encounter difficulty obtaining background information because of resistance of the examinee to consent, or resistance of the third party to provide the information. Limited access to the information may spring out of good intentions of the resistant third party. For example, in an attempt to safeguard health care information, providers may claim that the Health Insurance Portability and Accountability Act (U.S. Department of Health and Human Services, 1996) prohibits the release of certain records and that the requested records exceed what is "minimally necessary." In other instances, a key collateral source of information may be difficult to reach. The extent to which psychologists should strive to satisfy due diligence in the pursuit of background information is difficult to define. The psychologist is advised to make multiple attempts and to clearly document the process. When a critical piece of data is not obtainable, it may be necessary to halt, temporarily or altogether, the completion of the evaluation. Once an effort has been initiated to obtain data, it is difficult to make the case that the data, should they prove difficult to obtain, were not really essential to the evaluation.

Is it appropriate for psychologists to use the Internet to investigate an examinee's background? There are a number of issues to be considered in making this determination (Grote, 2004). It could be argued that it is not only appropriate, but necessary, for the psychologist to make use of publicly available information to provide a fully informed opinion. To what extent can, or should, the psychologist personally investigate the background of the examinee? Although the answer to that question may depend on the professional context, the most responsible course of action may be for the examiner to notify the examinee beforehand that such a review may be performed. The decision of whether to pursue the examinee's consent in this context is complicated by the fact that if consent is denied, the psychologist may have less access to certain aspects of the examinee's background than does the general public (Grote, 2004).

Depending on the nature of the evaluation, the examinee may not have the right to withhold consent. Given the complexities of the legal situation, it is always worthwhile to make the referral source aware of such hurdles to the evaluation; doing so often resolves the issue.

IMPARTIALITY

Competent and objective forensic psychologists attempt to ensure the accuracy of the information they obtain. To do so, they frequently look beyond documents and pursue additional sources of information. Individuals who know or have interacted with the examinee are one such source of information. Collateral sources are often able or willing to convey more during a personal contact than through written documentation. For example, consider the case of a 58-year-old married man who sustained a very minor work-related head injury. During an evaluation 8 months after his injury, he stated that he had not been able to read since his injury. He gave consent for a number of individuals to be contacted, including his wife. During the course of a telephone interview, his wife related that they both began each morning by reading the newspaper, aspects of which they typically discussed. Such information can be extremely valuable when making a determination regarding the validity of the examinee's statements and responses.

It is important to obtain informed consent from the collateral sources of information, in addition to that provided by the examinee. Consistent with ethical principles of autonomy, nonmaleficence, and justice, individuals serving as collateral sources of information are typically entitled to know (a) the lack of confidentiality of their communications, (b) the psychologist's need to cite them as the source of the information provided, (c) the potential range of foreseeable consequences of the evaluation, and (d) potential foreseeable consequences of the information that they are providing. Failing to provide sufficiently detailed information about the nature of the interview or "tricking" the person into revealing information that may harm the examinee, whom they may wish to help, is not consistent with ethical practice. Some examiners choose to obtain information from collateral sources in writing, a practice that emphasizes the professional nature of the communication, thus reducing the potential for the collateral source to feel tricked. That procedure would likely rob the evaluator of some spontaneously shared data but would lessen the possibility of the third party feeling misled or manipulated.

The accuracy of the information provided by the collateral source, like that provided by the examinee, is subject to bias. In the scenario described earlier, imagine that the examinee's wife had supported his invalid contention that he could no longer read. The evaluator relying on that third-party information as incrementally increasing the validity of the findings would be making an error that would reduce the accuracy and utility of the assessment. Use of the multisource, multimethod strategy by a psychologist with a critical approach to all information obtained may help to increase the likelihood that the psychologist's conclusions will accurately capture the examinee's status relevant to the legal issue under investigation.

CASE 2: BACKGROUND INFORMATION IN CRIMINAL CASES

A prosecuting attorney refers a criminal defendant charged with bank robbery to a psychologist for an evaluation of the man's sanity at the time of the alleged offense, which was 1 month previous. The attorney highlights the fact that during the arrest, once the defendant's Miranda rights were read, the defendant stopped talking and asked for an attorney. This behavior, the attorney believes, clearly reveals "savvy awareness of his right to remain silent." The investigative material that is obtained includes the arrest documentation, which described the defendant as talkative and speaking in a rational but nervous manner when apprehended by the police. Police interrogation summaries reveal that the defendant was silent after he was told of his rights. Surveillance cameras clearly document the examinee robbing the bank.

During the clinical interview, the defendant presents as oriented and rational, although he is mildly suspicious. He denies hallucinations, and no delusions are elicited. He notes he has been in the state hospital on more than one occasion with a diagnosis of schizoaffective disorder and had, in fact, been released 1 month prior to the alleged bank robbery, following which he has been living at home with his elderly mother. He does not believe he has a mental disorder but describes a long history of methamphetamine use. When asked about the alleged robbery, he says he robbed the bank because "that was where the money was," and he needs more money to buy methamphetamine.

The evaluator contacts the district attorney and informs him that she needs the records of prior state hospitalizations. The attorney says that would take considerable time, and he is dealing with a strict timeline on this case. He says he needs the report very quickly to stay within legal guidelines. The psychologist is torn between her commitment to conducting an adequate evaluation based on sufficient background information and her desire to satisfy the time demands of the referral source. Ultimately, she agrees to provide the report without the benefit of the requested records.

Analysis

Identify the Problem

The psychologist provided an opinion regarding a criminal defendant's past mental state without completing a reasonably thorough review of background information relevant to the determination. It was appropriate to review investigative material, because this information is often the best source for reconstructing mental states during the time of a crime, but additional highly relevant information was potentially available. The psychologist recognized that such information was needed, and in fact requested it, but was ultimately willing to provide an expert opinion based on insufficient data. She based much of her forensic opinion on two factors—the defendant's current mental state and his having remained silent when read his rights on the day of the robbery.

Consider the Significance of the Context and Setting

The psychologist insufficiently attended to the fact that she had been retained as a partisan expert (Standard 3.07, Third-Party Requests for Services). Although she might have been right in assuming that the referring attorney would not intentionally withhold information from her, she should have also recognized the strong situational press for her to provide an opinion favorable to the referring side, in this instance the government. The context of the evaluation added weight to the pressure exerted by the prosecutor; that is, the psychologist perceived the entire legal system to be frustrated awaiting her report. Such pressure weighed heavily in her decision to provide an opinion absent necessary records.

Identify and Use Ethical and Legal Resources

The psychologist has a responsibility to provide forensic services consistent with the highest standards of the profession (SGFP II, A, Responsibility). The multisource, multimethod model of forensic evaluation requires reliance on as much relevant information from varied sources as is reasonably available. Failure to obtain and consider pertinent information, as was being considered in this case, may result in substantial harm to the defendant and society and is inconsistent with the principle of nonmaleficence (General Principle A, Beneficence and Nonmaleficence; Standard 3.04, Avoiding Harm).

The psychologist recognized her need to review records from psychiatric hospitalizations, particularly the most recent hospitalization, as this would give a clearer indication of the defendant's mental state just prior to the robbery (Standard 9.01, Bases for Assessments), but she felt considerable time pressure from her referral source. It is incumbent on forensic psychologists to "take special care to avoid undue influence upon their methods, procedures, and products, such as might emanate from the party to a legal proceeding" (SGFP VI, C, Methods and Procedures).

The psychologist realized that she could benefit from consultation with a colleague. She called two senior forensic psychologists that she had recently met at a workshop.

Consider Personal Beliefs and Values

At the time of entry into forensic work, the psychologist began to examine her personal views about the criminal justice system and the various parties in legal proceedings. In the context of this case, she again examined her views regarding those who are mentally ill, those who abuse substances, and those who perform criminal acts. She believed that she maintained no biases toward, or against, any of the parties. She believed that she was able to remain fair in evaluating information gained from the multisource, multimethod model and to provide balanced, reasonable testimony when called to do so (SGFP VII, D, Public and Professional Communications).

Develop Possible Solutions to the Problem

After reviewing the relevant ethical and legal references and consulting with colleagues, the psychologist considered several courses of action: (a) tell the district attorney that she could not provide an opinion without the hospital records; (b) write a report stating the tentative opinion at which she had already arrived; she knew she could always change her opinion if new and important information became available; and (c) write a report, indicating that the results were "preliminary" and pointing out the missing portion of her formulation and the potential impact that information might have on her opinion.

One of the colleagues she had consulted had informed her that writing a report prematurely to satisfy the urgency of the referral source may indeed reflect prosecutorial bias, and that raised the concern that such bias might affect her opinions. Based on that frank feedback, she engaged in renewed self-examination of her values.

Choose and Implement a Course of Action

Given the pressure to produce a report that might be helpful to the court, she decided to write a preliminary report, which outlined her evaluation methods, results, and opinions. This report also disclosed the fact there was information not reviewed that, once available for review, might prove quite important in the clinical and forensic opinion formulations. She believed that by making her report preliminary and disclosing the limits of her expert opinion she was complying with the aspirational goal set forth in the SGFP (VI, H, Methods and Procedures), indicating that the forensic psychologist should limit expert opinions when the scope of the evaluation is not fully adequate to provide that opinion. It could be argued, however, that reaching a preliminary opinion, without all of the necessary data, is precisely a failure to achieve this goal. Even though the report is designated preliminary, it clearly reflects the bias or leaning of the evaluator, who may have a hard time convincing others that she remained receptive to the forthcoming information, particularly if that information did not result in a change of stance.

Assess the Outcome and Implement Changes as Needed

The forensic evaluator provided the preliminary opinion in written form to the district attorney as requested. Later, during testimony, she reiterated the limitations of her opinion given the limited informational sources. The judge then provided additional time for her to complete a more thorough evaluation, which included a review of the medical records and an interview of the defendant's mother. The psychologist, upon incorporating the additional information, was then able to testify with more certainty regarding her clinical and forensic conclusions.

In retrospect, she realized there had been no need for her to provide a preliminary report and that it would probably have been preferable not to do so. She realized that the greater potential for harm came from providing a preliminary report with unsubstantiated conclusions than from waiting for additional information to arrive. When later discussing the outcome with one of the colleagues whom she had consulted, she was informed that she had been vulnerable to legitimate attack by the defense attorney and the fact finder and was fortunate to have escaped such an attack. Although the psychologist's involvement in this case was concluded, at least for the time being, the psychologist was convinced of the importance of avoiding being pressured into prematurely offering opinions in the future.

4

THE EVALUATION

The forensic evaluation typically involves gathering information, through a variety of means, about the clinical characteristics of the examinee that are relevant to the forensic issues of concern (Heilbrun, 2001). However, prior to performing a clinical interview or administering psychological tests, the examiner must establish with the examinee a mutual understanding of the purpose and nature of the evaluation, including limits on confidentiality, reporting of results, and possible uses of the findings. Depending on the context in which the evaluation is performed, the psychologist must obtain informed consent or assent from the examinee or a legal representative or, in the context of court-ordered evaluations, provide notification of the purpose of the evaluation (Standards 3.10, Informed Consent, and 9.03, Informed Consent in Assessments, of the American Psychological Association's [APA's] Ethics Code, 2002).

The right of the examinee to understand the nature and purpose of the evaluation is based on the fundamental right of individuals to freedom of choice. Freedom of choice underlies the ethical principle of autonomy. When the legal system has already limited the examinee's rights, the only choice for the examinee may be to undergo the evaluation or experience a negative consequence. To the extent that the examinee's ability to understand the information is limited because of intelligence, cognitive impairment, psychiatric state, or some other condition, surrogate decision making may be required. The need to impart to the examinee or the surrogate decision maker information about the evaluation, through the process of informed consent or assent, is established by statute in most jurisdictions as well as by standards and codes governing professional practice, and thus appears to be an established principle of mental health assessment (Heilbrun, 2001).

THE PSYCHOLOGIST–EXAMINEE RELATIONSHIP

The nature of the relationship between the psychologist and the examinee, and the manner in which the relationship is established, have significant implications for the validity of the information that is obtained and the value of the psychological opinion for the court. As part of the process of informing the examinee of the purpose and nature of the forensic evaluation, the psychologist has an ethical obligation to inform the examinee that a traditional doctor–patient relationship does not exist (Bush & National Academy of Neuropsychology [NAN] Policy & Planning Committee, 2005). Even absent this traditional doctor–patient relationship, the forensic examiner has ethical obligations to the examinee: The examinee should understand the nature and limitations of confidentiality, feedback, and treatment. An examination of these elements of the evaluation process follows.

INFORMED CONSENT, ASSENT, AND NOTIFICATION OF PURPOSE

Individuals to be examined or evaluated by the forensic psychologist have a fundamental right to understand the evaluation process and its potential implications (APA Ethical Standards 3.10, Informed Consent, and 9.03, Informed Consent in Assessments; Standards for Educational and Psychological Testing [SEPT; American Educational Research Association, APA, & National Council on Measurement in Education, 1999] Standard 8.4), including "their legal rights with respect to the anticipated forensic service" (Specialty Guidelines for Forensic Psychologists [SGFP; Committee on Ethical Guidelines for Forensic Psychologists, 1991; IV, E, Relationships). It is generally not sufficient for psychologists to know that informed consent must be provided; they must know what information to convey and when and how it should be conveyed.

Informed consent requires that the decision to participate in the evaluation is made in a "knowing, intelligent, and voluntary way" (Heilbrun, 2001, p. 70). The psychologist must define the parameters of the service to be provided and clarify the examinee's expectations. The information must be tailored to the specific legal context. With the exception of court-ordered examinations, the examinee has the right to provide partial consent; that is, to consent only to some aspects of the evaluation and reporting process. When partial consent is offered, the psychologist may wish to explore and address the examinee's concerns, but the psychologists ultimately will determine whether to conduct the evaluation in the face of such limitations.

When the examinee appears to lack the capacity to provide informed consent, the psychologist provides notice to the legal representative (SGFP IV, E2, Relationships), provides the examinee with an appropriate explanation, and seeks the examinee's assent (Standard 3.10b, Informed Consent). In situations in which the examinee's legal representative objects to the examination, the psychologist should notify the court and respond as directed (SGFP IV, E2).

When psychological services have been ordered by the court and there is not meaningful choice about participation, psychologists provide *notification of purpose*, which includes informing the examinee of the purpose and nature of the evaluation and the limits of confidentiality (Standard 3.10c, Informed Consent; SEPT Standards 8.4 [Comment] and 12.10). If the examinee is unwilling to proceed after thorough notification has been provided, "the examination should be postponed and the psychologist should take steps to place the client in contact with his/her attorney for the purpose of legal advice on the issue of participation" (SGFP IV, E1, Relationships).

To maximize the potential for understanding, the psychologist should provide information in language that is reasonably understandable to the examinee (Standards 3.10a, Informed Consent, and 9.03b, Informed Consent in Assessments; SEPT Standard 8.4 [Comment]); that is, the language should generally be appropriate to the language fluency, developmental level, and cognitive capacity of the examinee. The psychologist must ensure that the examinee understands the information that has been provided about the nature and purpose of the evaluation (American Bar Association, 1989). To verify that the information was understood, the psychologist should question the examinee about the concepts conveyed. Questions that require the examinee to paraphrase the examiner's wording or apply it to the examinee's specific context or to hypothetical contexts may be of value in determining the examinee's level of understanding (Heilbrun, 2001). The information should be repeated as needed to facilitate understanding. In addition, the most salient aspects of information should be reviewed at the beginning of each separate evaluation session. Guidelines and measures for assessing competence to consent to treatment (e.g., Appelbaum & Grisso, 1995; Grisso, 2003; Grisso & Appelbaum, 1998a, 1998b) may apply in forensic settings as well (Heilbrun, 2001).

When information related to informed consent or notification of purpose does not seem to have been fully understood, the psychologist must determine whether the understanding obtained is sufficient to continue with the examination. Consultation with the examinee's attorney may help to clarify whether it is in the best interests of the examinee and the court for the examination to proceed. Depending on the context, the consent of a surrogate decision maker may be required. The steps in this process should be clearly documented (Standard 3.10d, Informed Consent).

Obtaining Assent of Minors

Jurisdictional statutes define the age at which one is legally able to make decisions independently, although the age may differ within jurisdictions depending on the issue being decided. Typically, individuals under 18 years of age are considered minors with respect to providing authorization for psychological services. As a result, authorization from one holding the legal right to consent to the evaluation on behalf of the minor is usually required. Such authorization may be provided by a custodial parent, court order, or other legal surrogate decision maker, such as an attorney, depending on the circumstances (Heilbrun, 2001). In addition, the cooperation of the minor should be sought. Both the legal representative and the minor must be informed, in developmentally appropriate language, of the purpose and nature of the evaluation, the potential uses of the information that is obtained, and potential consequences of refusal to cooperate. Their understanding of the information should be determined, and an assent form may be valuable for documenting that all parties understood the purpose and nature of the evaluation process at the outset.

Limits of Confidentiality

A primary difference between forensic and clinical psychological services is the nature of confidentiality. With some exceptions, communication between patient and doctor in a clinical context is protected. The APA Ethics Code states that protecting confidential information is a primary obligation of psychologists (Standard 4.01, Maintaining Confidentiality). In contrast, communications made in a forensic context are generally subject to review by others and, in many instances, may become a matter of public record. Forensic psychologists must discuss all foreseeable disclosures with the potential examinee or his or her legal representative as part of the consent–notification process. After advising the examinee of the potential uses of the examination findings, the psychologist should not disclose results or findings in another context without explicit informed consent to do so (SGFP IV, E3, Relationships).

Feedback

In many clinical settings and in some forensic contexts, psychologists provide examinees with feedback about the results of the evaluation. In situations in which feedback will not be provided, the examinee is notified of this fact at the outset the evaluation (Standard 9.10, Explaining Assessment Results).

PROCEDURES AND MEASURES

The APA 2002 Ethics Code states, "Psychologists base the opinions contained in their recommendations, reports, and diagnostic or evaluative statements, including forensic testimony, on information and techniques sufficient to substantiate their findings" (Standard 9.01a, Bases for Assessments). Determining which techniques are sufficient may be challenging in some cases, and there is room for difference of opinion, given the complexities of cases, the range of assessment instruments available for consideration, and circumstances that might affect access to relevant materials or collateral resources.

The assumptions, roles, and alliances inherent in forensic practice necessitate the use of a comprehensive evaluation methodology, consisting of systematic incorporation of multiple data sources (Denney, 2005; Heilbrun, 2001; McLearen, Pietz, & Denney, 2004; Melton, Petrila, Poythress, & Slobogin, 1997; Mrad, 1996; Shapiro, 1991). Typically, the forensic psychological evaluation consists of the following procedures: Review of records, interviews with collateral sources of information, behavioral observations, interview(s) with the examinee, and psychological testing. Because review of records and interviews with collateral sources were discussed in previous sections, the focus of this section is on behavioral observations, interview(s) with the examinee, and psychological testing.

Behavioral Observations

Behavioral observations may occur within or beyond the evaluation room, depending on the psychological questions being asked and the hypotheses being considered. Observations that occur across settings on multiple occasions may help to maximize the reliability of the information obtained from the behaviors being observed. A multisource, multimethod approach increases the likelihood of making accurate assessment of consistencies between behavior and self-report (Shapiro, 1999). Establishing a pattern of consistency adds confidence to the diagnostic formulation or helps reveal disingenuous claims.

In certain circumstances, tremendously meaningful information can be gained through surreptitious observation. In settings such as correctional centers and hospitals, observations made of the examinee when the examinee is not aware of the observation are often readily available from correctional officers and nursing staff. Even in the private practice setting, it takes little effort to observe, for instance, the examinee walking to his car and entering the driver's seat after he just informed you that he can no longer drive because of his disability. However, consistent with the principle of autonomy, the examinee has a right to be informed during the consent process that data from such observations may be obtained and considered.

Investigative information in criminal cases often includes audio and video recordings of defendant behavior at the time of an alleged offense, and it is competent practice to incorporate that information in the formulation of past mental states (Denney & Wynkoop, 2000). It is also not unusual to have available video surveillance of plaintiffs in personal injury cases or insurance disability cases. Using such information in evaluations may seem inappropriate to some clinicians, but in forensic mental health evaluations, by contrast, reliance on a variety of data sources is the standard of care, and litigants are informed at the outset that corroboration of claims will be sought.

The forensic evaluator bears the burden of ensuring that any such material reviewed is admissible in a court of law. To review, and therefore to potentially rely on, material that was illegally obtained may render the evaluator's findings and conclusions inadmissible. For that reason, it is prudent to ask that all information provided be scrutinized by the retaining attorney (or, when the evaluation is being performed by court order or agreement of the parties, such as might occur in an assessment concerning contested parenting issues, by all attorneys to the matter) to be sure that it is appropriate for review. It is also essential to maintain copies of any such material reviewed so that the data on which conclusions were based can be provided, if necessary, in response to challenges.

An evaluation of a criminal defendant in the correctional environment under court order establishes limitations on examinee privacy. One case illustrated that review of recorded telephone conversations made during the evaluation can verify the presence of exaggerated deficits (Wynkoop & Denney, 1999). The fact the tapes were relied on in the evaluation was reviewed by the U.S. district judge overseeing the case, and their use was not considered a violation of the defendant's right to privacy in that instance. Because the defendant was housed in a correctional facility for the evaluation and was specifically warned that his behavior during the evaluation period was not private, and because placards were placed next to the inmate phones indicating they were subject to review, the court viewed there to be no constitutional concerns. Those facts also relieved the ethical concerns about reviewing surreptitious telephone conversations in this instance, in the authors' view (Wynkoop & Denney, 1999).

Interviews

Face-to-face or in-person interviews with the examinee are typically an essential aspect of the evaluation process. The examinee's thoughts, feelings, and memories are fundamental to the forensic issue at hand. However, the subjective nature of the examinee's experience and the potential for bias may reduce the reliability of information obtained from interviews. Sbordone, Rogers, Thomas, and de Armas (2003), in summarizing the literature on the accuracy of criminal defendants' autobiographical memory, stated that the primary problem with "utilizing a defendant's recollection of what occurred during the alleged crime is that their memory of this event is likely to change over time" (p. 479). Such change tends to be in the direction of decreasing their culpability. Similarly, Bieliauskas (1999) cautioned,

> It is important to be careful in obtaining the history of a patient directly from the patient himself or from relatives and friends. On the face of it, these individuals should know the patient's situation best. . . . However, it is also the case that the veracity of interview information is open to question in forensic evaluation. (p. 125)

Williams, Lees-Haley, and Djanogly (1999) reviewed the empirical research in personal injury evaluation and concluded that there was significant risk for distortion in symptom presentation, when a great deal may be at stake and pressures may exist causing the litigant to report in ways designed to help the legal case. They advised clinicians working in this area to adopt a more analytical, data-oriented attitude toward patients' self-reports when conducting forensic examinations than they might in working with people in more traditional clinical settings.

The capacities of children to accurately recollect events, benign or traumatic, have been vastly researched, and effective interview protocols have been recommended for forensic evaluators to follow to ensure that the most accurate and detailed possible information is gathered, without contamination (Ceci & Bruck, 1995; Ceci & Hembrooke, 1998; Kuehnle, 1996; Poole & Lamb, 1998; Saywitz & Snyder, 1996). In general, child interviews require an appreciation for the capacities of children to understand complex constructs and to express notions about time, source attribution, and causal relationships. Children may respond to interview characteristics differently from adults and may be somewhat more vulnerable to influences that may shape the nature or accuracy of their recollections.

Good data can be gathered from children by interviewers trained to do so, but the contours of this arena are not necessarily intuitively obvious, and specialized training is essential.

Psychological Testing

One of the strengths of psychological testing, as part of a psychodiagnostic evaluation, is the introduction of standardized measurement of cognitive and emotional functioning and personality organization, as contrasted to reliance on clinical judgment alone. Many commonly used psychological and neuropsychological measures were not developed for forensic purposes, however, and do not have relevant normative data. Standard 9.02b, Use of Assessments, states, "Psychologists use assessment instruments whose validity and reliability have been established for use with members of the population tested. When such validity or reliability has not been established, psychologists describe the strengths and limitations of test results and interpretation." The SEPT (Standards 12.5, 12.13, and 12.16) addresses this issue as follows: "Many tests measure constructs that are generally relevant to the legal issues even though norms specific to the judicial or governmental context may not be available" (p. 129); however, "if no normative or validity studies are available for the population at issue, test interpretations should be qualified and presented as hypotheses rather than conclusions" (p. 131).

This caveat does not mean that psychologists in forensic contexts should only use tests specifically developed or standardized on specific forensic groups, such as pretrial criminal defendants or children involved in family court. Rather, it highlights two important and related issues: (a) use of tests in unique populations and (b) the validity of the measured construct as an indicator of a specific functional legal ability.

First, forensic psychologists must recognize the uniqueness of the population from which the examinee comes (Standard 9.02, Use of Assessments). Forensic examiners are not required to only use tests developed and standardized on forensic populations, but they must be cognizant that a particular forensic setting may include an atypical population, a population that was underrepresented in the standardization sample. Obvious examples include age, education, race, and nationality, but other less obvious groups may include lower levels of intellectual functioning or lower socioeconomic status found in some forensic settings. In some situations, it may be helpful to develop local norms to better understand the sensitivity and specificity of unique findings in a particular population. This does not mean, however, that one must use an achievement test, for example, that was standardized in that exact forensic setting, because such instruments measure a general psychological ability.

The results of tests or indices that have been developed with one forensic population may not generalize to different forensic populations. Such tests or indices may require validation with different forensic populations before being broadly used. Consider, for example, the Fake Bad Scale (FBS; Lees-Haley, English, & Glenn, 1991) of the Minnesota Multiphasic Personality Inventory—2 (MMPI–2; Butcher et al., 1989). With personal injury populations, this scale has been found to be a sensitive indicator of somatic malingering apart from the standard MMPI–2 validity scales (Larrabee, 1998, 2003a, 2003b). However, it is not yet clear how the FBS performs with criminal forensic populations (Larrabee, 2005). In situations such as this, the forensic examiner should carefully consider appropriate use of the test or index and cautious interpretation of the results. Forensic examiners using the FBS with criminal populations should use qualified statements when describing the meaningfulness of elevated scores until additional research is completed.

The second issue involves taking a measured construct as an indicator of a specific functional legal ability without it having been validated as a measure of that ability. For example, a criminal defendant with an above-average IQ score is not necessarily competent to stand trial simply because he has an above-average IQ. There are specific instruments developed to measure the specific legal function of competency in this regard. However, most clinical psychological tests have not been validated as measures of specific legal abilities, even though many have a logical and face valid relationship to at least part of the legal construct. Forensic examiners need to proceed with caution when extrapolating results of general clinical assessment instruments to specific legal questions. When such extrapolation occurs, forensic examiners are best served by providing interpretations that are qualified or presented as hypotheses rather than conclusions. However, it is not sufficient to merely state that caution was used in the test interpretation. Although stating that the results were interpreted with caution may alert the reader to a lower level of confidence in the findings, the examiner should specifically state the manner in which deviations from standardized testing conditions or normative samples may have impacted the test results or interpretation.

In addition to the considerations of nomothetic (norm-based) methods and evidence described previously, forensic examiners typically use ideographic (case-specific) data (Heilbrun, 2001). The value of considering the relevance of ideographic data for a specific examinee is understood by most examiners and, because of their face validity, may be particularly relevant to issues before the court and may, even absent the scientific rigor of other types of validity, carry considerable weight with a trier of fact (Grisso, 2003). Heilbrun (1992) identified criteria that should be addressed in the selection of a test instrument that is to be used in forensic assessment to ensure the relevance and accuracy of conclusions derived from such testing. First, the instrument should be commercially available with both a manual, describing adequate psychometric properties, and a review in *The Mental Measurements Yearbook* (Buros Institute of Mental Measurements, Lincoln, Nebraska) or another readily available source of relevant information. Second, a test whose reliability coefficient is less than .80 should be used only with explicit justification. Third, the test should bear relevance to the legal issue or its underlying construct, as evidenced in research published in refereed journals. Fourth, administration should follow standardized procedures designed to provide, as nearly as possible, a distraction-free setting. Fifth, population and situation specificity should be considered in the interpretation, with the examiner's confidence in the applicability of the results calibrated to reflect the closeness of fit. Sixth, objective tests and actuarial data, demonstrably relevant, are preferable to clinical observation. Seventh, response style should be assessed by methods sensitive to distortion and interpreted in the context of that response style. This focus on relevance and reliability in test selection will assist the psychologist working in a forensic setting to meet the demands of legal decision makers regarding admissibility and usefulness of their opinions.

Symptom Validity Assessment

Forensic evaluations must include assessment of the validity of the examinee's symptoms and presentation, to determine whether the examinee may be engaging in impression management. Even with those individuals for whom standardized testing is not appropriate (e.g., because of severe behavioral problems, apparent severe cognitive impairment, acute psychosis), the validity of the individual's presentation should be assessed through other evaluation methods, such as behavioral observations, interviews of collateral sources, and review of records. Such evaluation methods may reveal inconsistencies in the examinee's presentation that suggest volitional or psychiatric fabrication or exaggeration of symptoms. Additionally, invalid symptom manifestation may reflect irrelevant or uncooperative behavior (Heilbrun, 2001) or feelings of justification, entitlement, frustration, neediness, greed, or manipulation (Iverson, 2003).

Impression management may consist of either a posture of defensive denial of symptomatology (its absence or minimization) or exaggeration or feigning of symptoms. Current symptoms and symptom history each may be misrepresented. In forensic assessments in which the litigant has a vested interest in appearing virtuous or normal, the litigant may deny existing symptoms and present as "too good to be true." Litigants in contested parenting matters or fitness-for-duty assessment, for example, demonstrate a higher degree of defensive responding or other efforts at a distortion (Bagby, Nicholson, Buis, Radovanvic, & Fidler, 1999; Bathurst, Gottfried, & Gottfried, 1997; Siegel, 1996; Siegel & Langford, 1998). Although the assessment of potential minimization of symptoms is essential in some evaluation contexts, the assessment of exaggerated or feigned symptoms has been emphasized in the psychological literature in recent years and is the focus of the remainder of this section.

Symptom validity research has undergone tremendous growth in recent years, and the number of measures and indices of cognitive and psychiatric symptom validity has increased considerably. However, the explosion in symptom validity research and test development seems to have outpaced professional guidelines for their appropriate use. Although detailed review of symptom validity assessment is beyond the scope of this section, ethical concerns regarding symptom validity assessment are addressed below. Although thorough symptom validity assessment requires a multimethod approach, the focus of this section is on the selection, use, and interpretation of symptom validity tests (SVTs).

Differences in the approach to symptom validity testing, contrasted to other psychological testing, emerge at the outset of the evaluation. As part of the informed consent process, psychologists typically describe the methods and procedures that will be used during the evaluation. The degree of detail provided may vary considerably among psychologists. Some psychologists may provide information that measures will be used to assess the examinee's effort to do well, and even discuss the importance of being forthcoming and doing one's best, whereas others may mention this factor briefly or not at all. The extent to which detail is provided will reflect the degree of deception that the psychologist chooses to use in the evaluation (the issue of examiner deception is discussed in more detail below). Whatever tack is determined to be appropriate in disclosing this aspect of the forensic assessment, the evaluator should apply it consistently, providing the same information regardless of which party has requested the evaluation.

With symptom validity assessment, forensic psychologists may stray, unintentionally or intentionally, into areas of questionable ethical conduct. Unintentional ethical misconduct may result from insufficient competence in forensic practice or assessment; for example, the psychologist may fail to use some measure of impression management when the nature of the evaluation calls for it. Standard 9.01a, Bases for Assessments states, "Psychologists base the opinions contained in their recommendations, reports, and diagnostic or evaluative statements, including forensic testimony, on information and techniques sufficient to substantiate their findings." Psychologists bear the burden of justifying their selection of tools for evaluation, and the absence of SVTs or measures in forensic examination may be difficult to justify or may draw into question the adequacy of the assessment to substantiate the opinions offered.

Some of the recently developed SVTs have demonstrated sensitivity and specificity that exceeds that of measures on which psychologists relied a decade ago. Heilbrun (2001), noting that relatively few well-validated specialized measures exist, at least in some areas of forensic assessment, identified the use of testing to assess response style to be an emerging principle of forensic mental health assessment; however, considerable progress has been made with symptom validity testing in the past few years. It is incumbent on the forensic practitioner to maintain current knowledge of symptom validity research and instrumentation relevant to the practice area (Standards 2.03, Maintaining Competence, and 9.08, Obsolete Tests and Outdated Test Results).

In addition to inadvertent ethical misconduct related to competence, differences in symptom validity measurement selection, administration, interpretation, and use can lead to the appearance of intentional manipulation by the examiner to serve a specific purpose. Test selection may at times be guided, deliberately or unintentionally, by the examiner's wish to develop a certain result. Not all SVTs have equivalent sensitivity. An examiner wishing to give the appearance of testing symptom validity, but also to avoid detecting malingering or some other form of symptom invalidity, may select tests that have relatively poor sensitivity. The examiner may also administer the fewest number of measures that he or she believes can be justified. In contrast, an examiner wishing to demonstrate invalid symptom manifestation may administer a number of SVTs in the hope that at least one score will fall below an established cutoff. Psychologists engaging in either of these patterns of test selection give the appearance of intentional misconduct. In addition, examiners who differentially select the number and type of SVT depending on which side has retained them may have a particularly difficult time defending allegations of biased test selection.

The manner in which SVTs are administered may also be inappropriately manipulated to support a given position. For example, certain very simple measures of effort appear to assess memory (e.g., the Rey 15-Item Memory Test), and recommended instructions require the examiner to describe the measures as being difficult (Lezak, 1995). However, the extent to which the difficulty level is emphasized has the potential to influence the examinee's performance. Such manipulation of outcome may be difficult to detect. It is the ethical obligation of the forensic practitioner to use instruments fairly.

Interpreting SVT scores or patterns of scores, within the context of overall findings, poses perhaps the greatest opportunity for SVT misunderstanding and abuse. There is currently a dearth of professional guidelines available to assist the examiner. Although SVT practice guidelines have been developed for specific areas of psychological practice (e.g., Bush et al., 2005), additional SVT guidelines are needed for other areas of forensic practice. In the interim, it may be difficult for the examiner to know exactly what meaning to attribute to an SVT score or pattern of scores, and the biased examiner may abuse this ambiguity in SVT interpretation. For example, consider the following excerpts from a hypothetical neuropsychological report. The evaluation was performed following a clinical referral in the context of a disability claim and civil litigation 6 months after a work-related accident. The hypothetical report began as follows:

> A 60-year-old woman tripped and fell at work, hitting her knee and head. There was a brief loss of consciousness and a 24-hour period of posttraumatic amnesia. Her first memories consisted of medical interventions by hospital staff while on the neurology service. A CT scan of the brain was negative. The patient was discharged home to her husband's care 2 days after admission . . . The patient is a poor historian because of retrograde memory problems. She reported that she lost all memory from her childhood on. She reported that she only knows the information that she does know because her husband and childhood friends have reminded her of certain details.

The report included the following statements regarding symptom validity:

> Rapport was excellent, and the patient appeared to try her best. Thus, the results of the evaluation were considered to be a valid representation of the patient's cognitive, behavioral, and psychological functioning.

Later in the report, the examiner wrote,

> The results of symptom validity testing were equivocal. Although some results were within normal limits and others were below established cutoffs, none were significantly below chance.

The only SVT listed was the Rey 15-Item Memory Test, and no SVT scores were reported. Despite reporting invalid performance on some SVTs, the psychologist diagnosed impairments and their cause, localized cerebral dysfunction, and made a determination regarding disability:

> The patient presents with a variety of cognitive, behavioral, and psychological problems that emerged following a head injury that she sustained at work. The results of this preliminary examination suggest that some neurologic functions have been compromised by injury to the brain, with impairment of neurobehavioral and neurocognitive status resulting from damage to dorsolateral, orbital, and mesial prefrontal systems. The symptom picture and documented deficits are indicative of a totally disabling injury.

In the discussion section, the psychologist attempted to justify poor performance on SVTs:

> A complicating factor in this patient's case is her variable performance on measures of symptom validity. . . . Her performance in this area is equivocal, which makes interpretation of her cognitive abilities difficult. . . . Consideration has been given to the possibility that she has exaggerated her deficits. However, the pattern of findings is not consistent with exaggeration or fabrication of symptoms. The patient has consistently and vociferously emphasized her wish to return to her job. Despite the income received from Worker's Compensation, her financial situation has been negatively affected by her inability to work since her accident, creating a hardship for the patient and her family. . . . A more likely explanation for her variable performance on measures of symptom validity may be found in her severe attention problems. For those SVTs on which her performance fell below expectations for individuals with brain injuries, her performance was not below chance, which would be more reflective of malingering. Thus, the patient's variable performance on effort tests appears to reflect her severe difficulties with attention.

The examiner considered her potential for self-bias:

> Throughout the evaluation process, primary threats to examiner objectivity that may bias the interpretation of neuropsychological data were considered (Sweet & Moulthrop, 1999b), and a strong commitment to objectivity was maintained. As a result, this evaluation is considered to have been thorough and impartial.

Some may argue that the statements made regarding symptom validity reflect a reasonable point of view, given the lack of consensus within the field of psychology regarding the manner in which SVTs should be interpreted. However, the psychologist's justification of her test interpretation reflects, in our view, a lack of objectivity. In addition, use of the Sweet and Moulthrop (1999a) recommendations, although cited in the report, was not reflected in the psychologist's reasoning.

There may be legitimate difference of professional opinion regarding SVT use, and there are, as yet, few established professional directives. As a result, it may be difficult to determine in individual cases whether a practice reflects the best interests of justice or the best interest of the examiner's referral source, to the extent that those positions differ. Psychologists must determine for each case the appropriate selection, use, and meaning of indicators of response validity or bias to ensure the validity of examination findings. This thoughtful approach may ensure that the evaluation most effectively addresses the psycholegal question in a relevant and reliable way (Bush, 2004d).

As Blau (1998) stated, "The validity and reliability of expert opinion as to the presence or absence of malingering is a complex issue. . . . Testimony regarding malingering brings the expert close to being the Thirteenth Juror" (p. 19). To err by diagnosing malingering, when an alternative explanation for symptom invalidity may be present, "is essentially to accuse an individual of a potentially criminal act (e.g., fraud, perjury), while possibly also denying needed clinical services (e.g., treatment of depression)" (Sweet, 1999, p. 262). Therefore, psychologists have an affirmative obligation to conduct a thorough and objective evaluation of symptom validity and to consider and document all potential explanations for invalid symptom reporting or manifestation.

Examiner Deception

As mentioned previously, to some extent deception is required of the examiner in using SVTs. Psychologists may give general information suggesting that among the tests are measures of response style or validity, but they do not inform examinees that a specific measure (or index embedded in a specific measure) assesses the validity of their responding. Such information would invalidate the SVT or index. Thus, psychologists use deception to detect deception. Is this necessary, and is it ethical? The emerging standard of practice appears to support informing examinees, in the informed consent or notification of purpose process, that their effort and honesty will be assessed. However, the measures used and often their specific instructions rely on deception for their effectiveness. Measures that appear to assess cognitive ability and are described as measures of a certain cognitive ability, such as memory, may actually be measures of the validity of cognitive symptoms. Such deception on the part of the psychologist departs from the goal of obtaining fully informed consent.

Heilbrun (2001), in the context of discussing testimony, stated, "There is no place for deception in forensic mental health assessment" (p. 274). Although the APA Ethics Code addresses the use of deception in research (Standard 8.07, Deception in Research), it does not specifically address deception in assessment. Consistent with General Principle C (Integrity), psychologists generally seek to practice in a truthful manner; however, there may be instances in which deception may be justified to benefit consumers of psychological services. In such instances, psychologists must be mindful of the possible effects of deception on the sense of trust or the emotional state of the examinee or others involved in the case, and they should attempt to minimize potential adverse effects of such deception (Bush, 2004d). Having provided general information related to the inclusion of measures or indices of response validity during the informed consent process, the examiner has, in our opinion, met the obligation to honestly inform, and to properly obtain informed consent from, the examinee.

LEGAL CONSIDERATIONS IN METHODS SELECTION

Forensic psychologists select the methods and procedures they determine to be most appropriate to address the psycholegal question at hand. Such selection decisions are guided not only by the psychometric merits of the instrument or procedure, but also by the admissibility standards established by the court, because the court serves as gatekeeper for determining whether the psychologist's testimony will be allowed. To assist with the determination of admissibility of forensic psychological evidence, the court has historically relied on the standard of "general acceptance." That standard was established in *Frye v. United States* (1923), in which the Supreme Court established that the methods and procedures on which psychological determinations are made "must be sufficiently established to have gained general acceptance in the particular field" (p. 1014).

In 1993, the case of *Daubert v. Merrell Dow Pharmaceuticals, Inc.* refined the standard of admissibility of expert testimony in federal jurisdictions, by articulating that methods and procedures must not only have achieved general acceptance in the field to which they belong but also be relevant to issues at hand and must have demonstrated scientific reliability and validity in contributing to the conclusions of the expert. The *Daubert* decision extends beyond the measures used to include the nature of the reasoning on which the expert's conclusions rest, both of which must be grounded in scientific method. Thus, forensic psychologists should be prepared to defend their choices of methods and procedures and the reasoning that flowed from data collection to the opinion offered in court, on the basis of both general acceptance and scientific merit. The forensic expert must be prepared to illuminate the path that led from data to opinion, even if the court does not demand it; failure to do so falls below the standard of practice (Grisso, 2003; Heilbrun, 2001). Whether admissibility is governed by *Frye* (1923), *Daubert*, or some other standard, and whether there are challenges raised regarding admissibility of the testimony to be offered, psychologists practicing in forensic contexts limit opinions to those supported by data collected through procedures recognized in the field as legitimate.

MANDATED MEASURES

The psychologist maintains responsibility for conducting an examination adequate to answer the referral questions. It is the psychologist's responsibility to determine the procedures that compose an adequate examination in a given case. Retaining parties may make requests for psychologists to administer specific tests. If the psychologist believes that different, or additional, measures should be used than those requested, an attempt should be made to explain the reasoning behind the preferred measures and seek to establish an understanding with the retaining party of the importance of the psychologist making such test selection based on professional expertise (Bush & NAN Policy & Planning Committee, 2005). If the retaining party indicates that the measures preferred by the psychologist are allowable but will not be reimbursed, the psychologist must determine how to proceed in an ethically appropriate manner. Possible courses of action include administering the additional tests pro bono or refusing to perform the examination.

The psychologist is ethically obligated to document in the report any restrictions placed on selection of methods and procedures. The psychologist maintains responsibility for instrument or technique selection and should accept, modify, or reject recommendations on the basis of their appropriateness for a given examination (Bush & NAN Policy & Planning Committee, 2005).

There may be instances in which the psychologist is asked to provide the retaining party with a list of the examination measures in advance of the examination. To minimize the possibility of successful coaching of the examinee, the psychologist may elect to provide related but nonspecific information, such as a description of the neuropsychological domains to be assessed or a list of all measures at one's disposal, without stating specifically which measures will be selected for the evaluation in question (Bush & NAN Policy & Planning Committee, 2005).

THIRD-PARTY OBSERVERS

Interest in observing forensic psychological evaluations, other than for training purposes, is to ensure that the examinee receives an appropriate and competently performed evaluation and to ensure that the examinee is not asked legally objectionable questions. Thus, in personal injury litigation, it is often the plaintiff's attorney who has an interest in observing an evaluation conducted by a psychologist who has been retained by the defense. In criminal settings, the defense attorney may request observation of an evaluation performed by the prosecution's expert. Although motives of ensuring adequacy of psychological evaluation and protecting the examinee's legal rights may justify demanding presence of counsel or designees in the examination room, potential threats to the evaluation's validity must be considered.

Effects on Performance

The social psychology literature has demonstrated that people perform differently when being observed (Guerin, 1986). This phenomenon, referred to both as *social facilitation* and as *reactivity*, refers to a change in one's behavior when and because it is under observation (Russell, Russell, & Midwinter, 1992). Observation has been found to facilitate performance on easy tasks and inhibit performance on more difficult tasks (Green, 1983). In addition, studies on the effects of observers on psychological test results have revealed that examinees perform differently when observers are present. Specifically, performance on measures of attention, processing speed, and verbal fluency was found to be negatively affected when a significant other observed test administration, whereas motor and cognitive flexibility results were not significantly affected (Kehrer, Sanchez, Habif, Rosenbaum, & Townes, 2000). Similarly, performance on a measure of delayed memory was negatively impacted by a third-party observer, whereas motor performance was not (J. K. Lynch, 1997).

Further, the effects of third-party observers on test results appear to extend to the use of recording devices. Preliminary studies suggest that audio recording negatively affected verbal learning and recall but not motor performance (Constantinou, Ashendorf, & McCaffrey, 2002), and video recording negatively affected immediate and delayed memory performance but not motor performance or recognition memory (Constantinou & McCaffrey, 2003). Thus, studies indicate that both direct observation and indirect observation through recording devices may have an effect on psychological test performance. Such influences pose a threat to the validity and reliability of subsequent interpretation of test results.

Ethical Guidelines

The SGFP (VI, A, Methods & Procedures) state, "Forensic psychologists have an obligation to maintain current knowledge of scientific, professional, and legal developments" and "are obligated to use that knowledge . . . in selecting data collection methods and procedures for an evaluation" (VI, A). On the basis of current research, third-party observation during standardized testing appears to be inconsistent with appropriate data collection procedures.

The APA Ethics Code (Standard 9.02a, Use of Assessments) requires psychologists to use assessment techniques and instruments "in a manner and for purposes that are appropriate in light of the research on or evidence of the usefulness and proper application of the techniques." Psychologists also must "indicate any significant limitation of their interpretations" (Standard 9.06, Interpreting Assessment Results). On the basis of the available research in this area, the implication of Standards 9.02a and 9.06 appears at this time to be that psychologists who allow observation of evaluations must indicate that such observation likely had an effect on the information obtained and that if memory testing was performed, such observation likely had a negative effect on the results. The extent and nature of observer effects on any individual case would likely be unknown, and this should be indicated as well. In addition to the necessity of following standardized testing procedures, the Ethics Code mandate to maintain test security (Standard 9.11, Maintaining Test Security) would be violated by allowing nonpsychologists to observe test administration.

The position of the NAN Policy & Planning Committee (2000a) on third-party observers is that "Neuropsychologists should strive to minimize all influences that may compromise accuracy of assessment and should make every effort to exclude observers from the evaluation" (p. 380). The American Academy of Clinical Neuropsychology (AACN, 2001) makes a distinction between *involved observers* (e.g., an attorney) and *uninvolved observers* (e.g., psychology students and other health care professionals). The position of AACN is that "it is not permissible for involved third parties to be physically or electronically present during the course of an evaluation assessment of a plaintiff patient with the exception of those situations noted below" (p. 434). Exceptions include adults with extreme behavioral disturbances and children.

The SEPT states, "In general, the testing conditions should be equivalent to those that prevailed when norms and other interpretive data were obtained" (Standard 5.4 [Comment]). Most of the commonly used psychological tests were not standardized with third-party observers present. In fact, the Wechsler Adult Intelligence Scale—Third Edition (Wechsler, 1997) manual states, "As a rule, no one other than you and the examinee should be in the room during the testing" (p. 29).

Trained Observers

It has been suggested that use of a trained observer, such as a psychologist, would be permissible as part of the discovery process in litigated matters (Blase, 2003). A psychologist who is present on behalf of the examinee's attorney may be perceived by the examinee as a source of support in an otherwise adversarial situation. Green (1983) reported that the presence of an otherwise evaluative observer would be of future help to the subject served to reduce evaluation apprehension. After an extensive review of the social facilitation literature, Blase (2003) concluded that "advising examinees that a trained observer, either a person or a recording device, will be

present to observe the examiner, may have beneficial effect on those examinees anticipating a negative outcome" (p. 379). Blase described the need
for research designed specifically to further address this question.

In situations in which the observer was a psychologist, issues of test
security would not be of concern, and the psychologist would appreciate
the need to be unobtrusive. Although the presence of a psychologist observer
would still deviate from standardized procedures, the adversarial context
of litigation itself deviates from test standardization and may also affect
test performance.

Laws

Jurisdictional laws may require that, in some contexts, examinees be
allowed to record the evaluation or have an observer present. For example,
the New York State Worker's Compensation Board *Statement of Rights and
Obligations, Independent Medical Examinations* states that "the claimant has
the right to videotape or otherwise record the examination" and "has the
right to be accompanied during the exam by an individual/individuals of
his/her choosing" (Section 137 Workers' Compensation Law).

Similarly, the Florida Supreme Court explained, "When resort to an
[independent medical examination] is necessary by either party, the parties'
relationship is clearly adversarial, and a physician performing an IME should
be treated as the requesting party's expert witness . . ." (*Adelman Steel Corp.
v. Winter*, 1992). The court further explained in *U.S. Security Insurance
Company v. Cimino* (2000), "There is nothing inherently good or bad about
the credibility function of an IME. If there is no court reporter or other
third party present at the examination, however, a disagreement can arise
between the plaintiff and the doctor concerning the events at the IME . . ."
The court found that "absent a valid reason for denial, an insured is entitled
to have an attorney or videographer present at a physical examination."

Essential Use of Third Parties

In some instances, observers serve an important function in facilitating
the psychological evaluation. For example, interpreters may be needed when
the examiner is not fluent in the language of the examinee. When interpreters are needed, psychologists must first assess the potential biases or other
influences of proposed interpreters. Interpreters who may have a stake in
the outcome of the evaluation should be avoided. Once an appropriate
interpreter has been selected, the examiner must

> Obtain informed consent from the examinee to use that interpreter,
> ensure that confidentiality of test results and test security are maintained,
> and include in their recommendations, reports, and diagnostic or evalua-

tive statements, including forensic testimony, discussion of any limitations on the data obtained. (Standard 9.03c, Informed Consent in Assessments)

In addition to the use of interpreters, the presence of a third party may be indicated when evaluating small children, examinees with substantial behavioral problems, or when the purpose of the evaluation is to assess the interaction between two or more people. The request sometimes arises for a child's therapist to accompany the child in an interview or evaluation session to accommodate the child's need for a trusted ally in the room. Although there may be merit in allowing therapist attendance, the potential contamination of the therapist's presence on the child's presentation should be carefully weighed. The therapist is an advocate for the child, and possibly for a particular view of history constructed through their therapy sessions together, potentially regarding the very issues cogent to the evaluation. If the therapist is present, the child may feel compelled to stay true to the version of history constructed through the therapist's interpretative handiwork. A mutually agreed on neutral third party, such as a former babysitter or neighbor, might be a more benign alternative.

Conclusion

The issue of allowing a third party into the examination session is complicated. Persuasive arguments are offered both for and against such presence. In fact, the issue in forensic practice is not so much whether third parties should be allowed, but rather who and under what conditions (Martelli, Bush, & Zasler, 2003). When considering allowing third parties into the psychological evaluation setting, psychologists are cautioned to carefully consider the potential effects of the third party on the validity of the data and on test security. Parties requesting observation of an evaluation, whether the proposed observation is direct or indirect, should be educated about the potential effects of the observation on the conclusions drawn, and should also be warned that any potential effects must be reported.

When observers are permitted, the situation should be structured to minimize the intrusion, with clear ground rules established before the examinee is present. The ground rules might include the following: (a) The observer must remain silent except to say, in a neutral tone, that the evaluation session needs to be interrupted or ended (if such power to abort it does lie with the observer); (b) the observer is to be seated outside the field of vision of the examinee; (c) the observer may not discuss what was observed with the examinee during breaks, between interview sessions, or between the evaluation and trial; (d) the observer must maintain strict confidentiality not only about the examinee's disclosures but also about the questions asked; and (e) under what circumstances and to whom the observer may report. It may be useful to preestablish the rule that the observer will write a full description of the observation after the observation ends but before having an opportunity to discuss the observation with others and that the notes are discoverable by both sides at a time preestablished. Additionally, the examiner's report should include detailed and specific information about the observer's behavior and apparent influence, if any, and the potential effects of the observer on the data and the opinions offered. Deviations from standardized procedures and from ethical guidelines should be carefully considered and the advantages and disadvantages weighed.

CULTURAL DIVERSITY CONSIDERATIONS

Ethical challenges in the consideration of ethnic and cultural diversity pose considerable difficulty for psychologists, as they cut across practice settings, age ranges, and psychopathological conditions. These challenges are faced not only by psychologists representing dominant U.S. demographics but also by those psychologists who are members of the minority groups with whom they work, as many psychological measures were not developed with such variations in mind and were not standardized on diverse groups or specific populations (Bush, 2004c).

Psychological functioning is influenced by one's sociocultural background. Despite commonalities that exist among members of the same races, ethnic backgrounds, and cultures, considerable intragroup differences exist (Manly & Jacobs, 2002). Therefore, the psychological evaluation must include a thorough exploration of the examinee's unique racial and ethnic identity and cultural background. Failure to consider factors such as race, nationality, place of birth, immigration status, the level at which the culture of origin is maintained, perception of health care institutions and professionals, cultural factors in family roles and interactions, and significance of religious influences may result in significant misunderstanding of the examinee and an increased potential for error in psycholegal opinions. In addition, some of the traits and abilities assessed by psychologists may differ from those that are valued by members of different cultures, and the expression of certain traits and abilities may differ (Iverson & Slick, 2003; Manly & Jacobs, 2002). Furthermore, failure by examiners to consider their own feelings toward, and understanding of, members of different groups may also contribute to misunderstanding of the examinee's psychological functioning.

APA General Principle D (Justice) states that all individuals are entitled to access to and benefit from psychological services of equal quality. Psychologists must be proactive in ensuring that biases and limitations of competence do not interfere with the provision of their services. Standard

2.01b, Boundaries of Competence, requires sensitivity to the impact of culture, disability, and other diversity factors on one's professional competency. Knapp and VandeCreek (2003) state, "It is not an ethical violation to provide less optimal treatment to members of . . . any groups; it is only a violation if the knowledge that is lacking is essential for providing services" (p. 303).

Standard 9.02b, Use of Assessments, requires psychologists to use assessment instruments that have established validity and reliability for use with members of the population that the patient represents. In the absence of such validity or reliability, psychologists must describe the strengths and limitations of the test results and interpretation. Standard 9.02c states that psychologists should use measures that are appropriate given the patient's language preference and competence, unless use of an alternative language is relevant to the examination. However, many of the psychometric challenges faced in the assessment of racial or ethnic minorities are potentially insurmountable (Iverson & Slick, 2003). Neither conceptual nor metric equivalence has been established for many tests, including nonverbal tests, administered to ethnic minorities. Standard 9.06, Interpreting Assessment Results, requires psychologists to "take into account" the various factors that may affect the accuracy of their interpretations. However, because of the number of potentially invalidating factors, "in some situations, it is impossible to determine if the interpretations made by psychologists under these circumstances could be valid" (Iverson & Slick, 2003, p. 2078).

Standard 9.03, Informed Consent in Assessments, addresses, in three subsections, informed consent in assessments relevant to cultural diversity. Standard 9.03c describes the need for psychologists to obtain informed consent before using the services of an interpreter. Determinations regarding the need for and selection of interpreters are challenging, and universal conclusions cannot be provided, but some general guidelines are suggested within the APA Ethics Code and can be expanded. The SEPT also provides guidelines for the use of interpreters: "When an interpreter is used in testing, the interpreter should be fluent in both the language of the test and the examinee's native language, should have expertise in translating, and should have a basic understanding of the assessment process" (SEPT, Standard 9.11). To be fully informed, the examinee should be told that the translation may result in a degree of imprecision in the test results, and the degree of imprecision will be greater the more divergent the dialect or regional variation of the language of the interpreter and the examinee. Standard 9.03c also outlines the responsibility of psychologists to ensure that their interpreters follow requirements to maintain confidentiality of test results and maintain test security.

The sections of the APA Ethics Code that address assessment issues consistently emphasize the need to state the limitations of one's interpretations and opinions, and culture, ethnicity, or use of interpreters potentially creates limitations. Standard 9.06, Interpreting Assessment Results, specifically states that linguistic and cultural differences must be appropriately considered when interpreting assessment results. Psychologists are expected to indicate any significant limitations of their interpretations. It is not sufficient to state that test results were interpreted with caution. The potential impact of linguistic and cultural factors must be described with as much specificity as possible. When measures are used that have not been standardized on the population of which the examinee is a member, interpretations should include a statement that the test results may misrepresent the examinee's true psychological state. When cognitive tests lacking adequate standardization with the specific population have been administered, the likely underrepresentation of the examinee's true ability should be stated.

Forensic examinees are often, at least for purposes of the forensic evaluation, in a class of vulnerable individuals who may have little capacity to exercise vigilance over the manner and quality of treatment they receive. The impact of the evaluation may, however, be of grave significance, and in the most extreme case may be a matter of life or death. In evaluations to assist in sentencing determinations for capital offenders, for example, the examinee is a member of a population of individuals known to have been exposed to extraordinary violence and brutalizing experiences, poverty, substance abuse, underemployment, and other factors that would be expected to shape the person's psychological functioning (Connell, 2003; Cunningham & Reidy, 2001). Norms for most or all psychological tests are unavailable for the population of incarcerated individuals facing capital murder charges. Although standardized testing may provide increased richness and depth in conceptualizations of the defendant's cognitive and behavioral styles and may provide for systematic comparison with norm groups, the use of such instruments in this setting may arguably be ethically inappropriate (Cunningham & Reidy, 2001). Not only are tests not normed for the population, but also the inferences drawn from test results may be more prejudicial than probative of the issue under consideration, focusing on the almost certain character pathology without consideration for "aging out" potential relevant to the question of release in 40 years, for example, contrasted to death (Cunningham & Reidy, 2001). Not so clearly identified as a culturally divergent population, this group of individuals may be subjected to unjust application of psychological expertise and instrumentation without concern for the ethical conflicts such application may raise.

Beyond test instruments, the evaluation is composed of other techniques of data collection, and cultural diversity may impact sharply on the nature of the data gathered and their interpretation in each of those areas. Cunningham and Reidy (2001) discussed the unique considerations that may be relevant in interviewing collateral contacts, particularly the defendant's family members, in a forensic evaluation of a capital defendant for sentencing. Subcultural variations in speaking to outsiders about private family matters, in revealing history of domestic violence or substance abuse, shame about poverty, and other such factors may cause the family members to be incapable of providing accurate information, particularly if given only one opportunity to do so. Special effort may be required to ensure that the collateral contact understands the importance of providing an accurate picture of the background from which the defendant came, of being forthcoming about the defendant's early symptoms of difficulty and the relative availability or absence of effective tools for intervention, of the history of chemical dependency that may have influenced the defendant's behavior, and other such issues that may be reflexively denied or hidden. Multiple interviews, occurring over time and in the home or neighborhood of the collateral contact, may be necessary to overcome resistances borne of cultural issues. The uniqueness of these kinds of assessment and the potential gravity of the outcome warrant special consideration of cultural variations and particular emphasis of the limitations of the psychological techniques used therein (Cunningham & Reidy, 2001).

There are many challenges to obtaining valid evaluation results from members of ethnic or racial groups that differ from those on which the psychological measures used were developed and normed. However, with awareness of potential ethical pitfalls and ways to avoid them, forensic psychologists can make appropriate referrals or conduct evaluations and make appropriate statements about the results.

RECORD OR PEER REVIEWS

The majority of this chapter has focused on the psychological evaluation of individuals; however, psychologists practicing in forensic contexts may also be asked to make determinations about cases solely on the basis of an examination of records. These record or peer reviews often take one of two forms. First, psychologists may be asked to render opinions about the work product (e.g., methods used and conclusions drawn about a patient or an examinee) of colleagues, opinions that may impact the lives of those seen by colleagues. Second, psychologists may be asked to render opinions about individuals involved in a forensic matter based on reviews of records, without having personally evaluated the individuals. Psychologists who perform, or are considering performing, such reviews should consider the relevant ethical guidelines, including the changes between the 1992 and 2002 APA Ethics Codes.

The 1992 APA Ethics Code (APA, 1992) advised psychologists to "provide written or oral forensic reports or testimony of the psychological characteristics of an individual only after they have conducted an examination of the individual adequate to support their statements or conclusions" (Standard 7.02b, Forensic Assessments). The 1992 Ethics Code provided the following exception:

> When, despite reasonable efforts, such an examination is not feasible, psychologists clarify the impact of their limited information on the reliability and validity of their reports and testimony, and they appropriately limit the nature and extent of their conclusions or recommendations. (Standard 7.02c)

The 1991 SGFP (currently under revision) provide essentially the same advice (VI, H, Methods and Procedures).

The 2002 Ethics Code directly addresses the issue of record review and similar consultation: "When psychologists conduct a record review or provide consultation or supervision and an individual examination is not warranted or necessary for the opinion, psychologists explain this and the sources of information on which they based their conclusions and recommendations" (Standard 9.01c, Bases for Assessments). Thus, the 2002 Ethics Code considers record review performed in appropriate contexts with clear representation of the information on which opinions are based to be consistent with ethical practice.

CASE 3: CUSTODY ISSUES IN FAMILY LAW

A court-appointed child custody evaluator is in the midst of data collection in a case involving joint custodial parents of a 7-year-old girl. The mother, upon remarriage, has filed a motion with the court to give her sole custody, as this would allow her to decide the child's residency. She anticipates relocation to a city about 1,300 miles away, asserting that her best chance of gaining employment is in the distant city and that she and her new husband enjoy the idea of living there. The father counterfiles, asserting that the mother's alienation of the child from him has been growing since the divorce and has reached untenable proportions with the proposed move. He wants sole custody to be awarded to him, because he has demonstrated a better capacity to respect the other parent's role in the child's life. Each parent seeks full decision-making power.

The mother moves to the new location before the hearing, taking the child with her and enrolling her in school there. She is participating in the custody evaluation by traveling to the home jurisdiction. On the occasion of the mother's travel to the home jurisdiction for her first interview, she brings the child on the trip and reportedly readies the child for an interview, although she has been clearly informed that the child will not be seen by the evaluator until after her (and the child's father's) second or third appointment, likely some weeks in the future. She then reports that the child has been overcome by stress at the idea of the interview and has been hospitalized locally for medical observation and evaluation, a hospitalization that lasts throughout the several days that they are in the area.

Owing to the possibility that the child is being put under undue pressure and stress by her mother in preparation for her first interview with the evaluator, despite the evaluator's efforts to educate the mother regarding how to buffer her and when to begin to prepare her, and in what way, the evaluator considers altering standard office procedures for data collection. Specifically contemplated is the idea of making an unannounced trip to the mother's new home city and arranging to conduct at least the child's first interview there, with her mother having no forewarning and therefore less probability of arousing further such stress in the child as the interview time approaches.

Analysis

Identify the Problem

Because the contemplated plan to travel to the distant city and make an unannounced visit to interview the child composed a significant alteration in standard office procedure and had not been included in the initial description each parent was given about the nature of the assessment process, it potentially represented ethically questionable action. Clearly the effort was to circumvent the mother's opportunity to prepare her child for the evaluation, to avoid the apparent likelihood that her preparation would result in an emotionally trying ordeal for the child.

Consider the Significance of the Context and Setting

There was nothing perceived to be patently unethical about conducting an unannounced home visit in a custody evaluation, in that many psychologists routinely conduct such visits as part of their standard evaluation protocol. Given that it was not this evaluator's standard procedure, had not been listed in the informed consent process as a potential part of the evaluation, and would increase the length and cost of the evaluation, the evaluator considered it problematic. As it happened, the father was charged by the court to bear the entire cost of the evaluation and would not likely have objected to this additional expense. The evaluator would not, of course, consult him about this additional cost before making the trip, given that such consultation would clearly place the evaluator in collusion with him in planning a circumvention of the mother's parental authority.

Further context to be considered was found by examining the court order for the assessment. The court had ordered the parents to cooperate with whatever structure the evaluator determined would be appropriate in conducting the evaluation. It was assumed the court would have no quarrel with the evaluator's contemplated plan, given that its primary function was to spare the child potential unnecessary emotional stress.

A final consideration was that the implementation of this plan could be construed to represent a prejudgment by the evaluator of the mother's contribution to the child's earlier reported stress reaction, a judgment for which there was, as yet, inadequate basis. Although it seemed probable, given the depth and texture of the mother's first interview revelations, the evaluator's opinion about the likelihood was not fully formulated and suspended judgment was maintained.

Identify and Use Ethical and Legal Resources

Even though the evaluator was fairly sure there was no clear ethical or legal proscription to the unannounced home visit, or to the variation of data collection methods from case to case, it seemed prudent to review relevant documents with the contemplated action in mind, to see if any interpretation or guideline needed to be considered. A review of the APA Ethics Code, the court order for the evaluation, and the state board rules of practice provided, as expected, no strictures or other applicable guidance. The evaluator was free to choose whatever procedures of data collection appeared to be warranted in conducting the evaluation. Assuming the technique chosen was one for which there was scientific and professional support, and that the evaluator was competent to use it, there was nothing to bar its implementation.

The *Guidelines for Child Custody Evaluation in Divorce Proceedings* (APA, 1994) was also consulted. It was clear from this reading that the evaluator could select the methods to be used in conducting the evaluation. Further review of professional literature supported the importance of using parallel processes with each party in conducting the evaluation (Otto, Buffington-Vollum, & Edens, 2002).

Collegial consultation proved to be a most valuable resource. An experienced colleague offered the observation that the evaluator's plan stood to so significantly disregard the family system that its potential value would be overshadowed by the potential harm. The evaluator and her colleague considered the principles of autonomy and nonmaleficence. The principle of autonomy supported the right of the child's mother (as well as father) to be fully informed of all evaluation procedures and to prepare her family and her home for the evaluation. The colleague further pointed out that giving the mother her opportunity to do what she would do, as she responded to the structure of the custody evaluation, provided the evaluator with material essential to the process of developing an opinion. In the context of examining potential harmful influences, the possible emotional distress to the child was considered, as was the long-term harm that could result from an inappropriate custody determination. Consistent with the principle of nonmaleficence, the evaluator wished to minimize or eliminate both types of harm; however, she realized that she would need to weigh the potential extent of each type of harm and make a decision based on the cost–benefit ratio.

Consider Personal Beliefs and Values

The evaluator had to consider the possibility that the mother's general approach to shared parenting, including her seemingly casual decision to move to a distant location to satisfy her own needs or whimsy, at obvious cost to the father's involvement with the child, aroused reactions that were counter to the evaluator's ethical obligation to formulate opinion only after all data were collected. That is, the evaluator's personal values resulted in a prejudgment of the mother's possible contribution to the child's distress and threatened to color the evaluator's overall receptivity to the mother's position. Such values, in fact, appeared to be motivating the evaluator to alter standard evaluation procedures for reasons other than professional dedication to objective assessment.

The value of nonmaleficence is held dear by those attracted to the helping professions. Child custody evaluators, even those whose practice activities are limited to forensic evaluations and for whom the practice of psychotherapy is little more than a distant memory, may struggle with staying true to the role of evaluator, wishing at times to ease the distress of the litigant or child. There is a strong pull, when it appears a child is being harmed by the process of the evaluation, to step out of the role of evaluator and become an intervener.

Develop Possible Solutions to the Problem

The psychologist developed four potential solutions to her dilemma: (a) perform the unannounced visit to the mother's home as planned, with no visit to the father's home; (b) perform visits to the homes of both parents; (c) forgo, as she often did, home visits; rather, require all interviewees to come to her office; or (d) inform the parent(s) that a home visit would be added to the evaluation protocol, thus allowing the parent(s) some opportunity to anticipate it and to prepare. The psychologist also considered whether a report to the local child protective agency would be required, given the observation that the mother might have been emotionally abusive in her manner of ratcheting up the child's distress.

Choose and Implement a Course of Action

The primary question was whether to circumvent the mother's opportunity to prepare her child for the first interview, by making an unannounced home visit for the first interview. Suspended judgment was in order, and the evaluator did, indeed, maintain a posture of receptivity as to how the mother would prepare the child.

The psychologist determined that if the unannounced home visit were to occur to the mother's home, a similar one needed to be made to the father's home. Even though there were no allegations being made about the adequacy of the physical structures, and the evaluator would generally have conducted home visits only in a case in which there was basis for concern, the importance of even-handedness dictated the use of parallel procedures with the parents. The evaluator considered that performing unannounced home visits in this case could effectively short-circuit the evaluation process and potentially deprive the mother of her opportunity to properly or improperly prepare her child.

The lack of substantial basis for the belief that the mother had emotionally abused the child, or would emotionally abuse the child, in her manner of preparing her for the visit decided the issue. The evaluator made the decision to forego the unannounced visit in favor of the standard procedure, a scheduled in-office appointment. This plan would ensure the continuation of the standard evaluation protocol used by the evaluator, would protect the mother's autonomy in preparing her child for the first interview, and would avoid any perception of the evaluator having prejudged the mother.

Recognizing that the child might be hurt in the process, the evaluator determined that the forensic task was, in fact, evaluation and not child protection. Considering the potential for mother to emotionally abuse the child in her preparation, the evaluator recognized that there was insufficient support for that concern to warrant a referral to the child protective agency. Thus, the evaluator opined that the emotional discomfort to the child would be relatively short term and would be worth the longer term benefit of an appropriate and ethically based custody determination.

Assess the Outcome and Implement Changes as Needed

The child was brought for the first interview by her mother and was apparently reasonably well prepared. She seemed to be relaxed and comfortable, and although she displayed age- and context-appropriate anxiety, she was not distraught. Ultimately, the court determined that the mother would have sole custody but that the child should continue to have regular contact with her father. Domicile of the child was restricted to the contiguous counties of the court of jurisdiction. The child was told of this outcome by her mother in the evaluator's presence, outside the courtroom (where she had arranged to have the stepfather wait with the child, against advice of counsel). The child responded to the news, delivered as if it were news of a death in the family, with tremendous emotional distress.

Although it is necessary for anyone, including a child custody evaluator, to report abuse or neglect to the protective service agency, a distinction may legitimately be drawn when the possibility of abuse, particularly emotional abuse, is being explored as part of the family court matter. To prematurely conclude that there is enough evidence of abuse to warrant a referral to the child protective services agency would place one in the position of needing to consider recusing oneself from the evaluation matter, in that it could be argued that a determination has been made before all of the data have been collected. Thus, in cases in which there is unsupported allusion to the possibility of abuse, the evaluator may justifiably forgo reporting the possible abuse during the pendency of the evaluation; of course, this does not exempt the evaluator from the necessity to comply with mandated reporting requirements when the evaluator has reason to believe abuse is occurring, even when such reporting may indeed result in the evaluator having to recuse herself. The present matter, however, had to do with the evaluator perceiving there to be a possible risk of the mother unnecessarily heightening the child's emotional distress just before the child's interview and did not necessarily implicate the mother in an ongoing pattern of emotional abuse. This concern appeared not to rise to the level intended to be included in the ambit of mandated reporting statute.

Months after this matter was concluded, the evaluator learned that the mother, stepfather, and child had relocated, against court orders, to yet another location, 2,500 miles away, and ultimately the child's father gave up further efforts to be involved in his child's life. It appeared, then, that the model for resolving the potential ethical challenge served very well in this matter; human nature, on the other hand, served just as it often does in such matters, but modification of it is not within the purview of forensic psychology.

5

DOCUMENTATION OF FINDINGS
AND OPINIONS

Consumers of forensic psychological services have a right to expect and receive competent services. For services to be considered competent, the opinions offered must be based on "information and techniques sufficient to substantiate their findings" (Standard 9.01a, Bases for Assessments, of the American Psychological Association's [APA's] Ethics Code, 2002). The law requires that expert opinions provided, and the methods of data collection and reasoning on which they are based, be generally acceptable within the professional community (*Frye v. United States*, 1923) and be able to withstand scientific scrutiny (*Daubert v. Merrell Dow Pharmaceuticals, Inc.*, 1993). It is generally the documentation of one's work that allows a reviewer to determine whether the evaluation performed was relevant, reliable, and valid.

To enable review, psychologists have an ethical obligation to appropriately document and maintain records of their work (Standard 6.01, Documentation of Professional and Scientific Work and Maintenance of Records), and the documentation must be accurate (Standard 5.01b, Avoidance of False or Deceptive Statements). The Specialty Guidelines for Forensic Psychologists (SGFP; Committee on Ethical Guidelines for Forensic Psychologists, 1991) state,

> When forensic psychologists conduct an examination or engage in the treatment of a party to a legal proceeding, with foreknowledge that

their professional services will be used in an adjudicative forum, they incur a special responsibility to provide the best documentation possible under the circumstances. (VI, B, Methods and Procedures)

Determining the nature of documentation that is "sufficient to withstand scrutiny in an adjudicative forum" and "the best documentation possible" may be a difficult task. However, documentation that is linked to a competent evaluation and is of sufficient detail to allow an independent peer reviewer to arrive at similar conclusions or clearly identify how the conclusions in a report or testimony were reached would most likely withstand adjudicative scrutiny.

Documentation throughout the process of forensic evaluation or treatment is necessary to ensure that competent services are provided and to assist the legal decision maker. Following the provision of services, the availability of the documentation for reviewers helps to determine that competent services were provided. In addition, such documentation protects clients, the public, and the psychologist (APA, 1993; Barsky & Gould, 2002). The foreknowledge by the forensic psychologist that his or her records may be reviewed provides considerable incentive to ensure that all facets of the evaluation or treatment process are performed at the highest possible level of competence. Thus, maintaining appropriate records is consistent with the APA Ethics Code's General Principles A (Beneficence and Nonmaleficence) and D (Justice) and is an underpinning of competent forensic psychological services to which consumers have a fundamental right.

SCOPE OF INTERPRETATION

The integration of scientific data and reasoning is important for relevant and reliable psychological decision making (Heilbrun, 2001). Psychological conclusions of value to the trier of fact tend to be based on a combination of individualized (ideographic) and group-referenced (nomothetic) approaches to data interpretation. Information specific to the examinee is collected and compared with the performance of one or more groups of interest. Cognitive, psychopathologic, or behavioral data that differ from the comparison groups must be understood in terms of the individual's unique life circumstances, with an emphasis on variables that are known to affect such performances. Opinion based on reasoning that lacks either the ideographic or nomothetic approach is weakened. The APA Ethics Code states, "Psychologists' work is based on established scientific and professional knowledge of the discipline" (Standard 2.04, Bases for Scientific and Professional Judgments). An opinion that is not grounded in objective data and scientific principles may be insufficient to meet the requirements of this standard.

Legal decision making tends to be dichotomous in nature, with referral sources and triers of fact preferring definitive statements regarding diagnosis, proximal cause, and other determinations relevant to the forensic issues at hand. Requests or demands for definitive statements tend to be at odds with the more probabilistic statements that are generally acceptable to clinicians and to clinical referral sources (Koocher & Keith-Spiegel, 1998). There is risk in offering definitive statements in forensic contexts that would traditionally have been offered as statements of possibility in clinical contexts. Such statements may be seen as inaccurate or misleading, in violation of the APA Ethics Code (Standard 5.01, Avoidance of False or Deceptive Statements) and counter to professional specialty guidelines (SGFP VII, A and B, Public and Professional Communications). It is important for the psychologist, having conducted a thorough evaluation, to assert opinions as strongly as the data merits but also to describe the limitations of those opinions.

Psychological capacities are a component of many legal questions, and psychologists are often retained to evaluate and comment on such capacities. However, there may be occasions when the psychologist's opinion regarding the legal question itself is requested. Offering an opinion on the ultimate legal question threatens to invade the province of the court, because it is specifically the task of the trier of fact to make this determination. Psychologists who attempt to answer the legal question directly are vulnerable to overstepping the bounds of their expertise and to inducing their data to support opinion about moral, political, and community-value components not actually within the expertise of psychology (Heilbrun, 2001).

Although there is no prohibition against answering the legal question, FRE 704 (FRE, 1984) explicitly permitting it, with some specific exceptions, and ethical guidelines cautioning that opinions offered be supportable, Heilbrun (2001) did identify as an emerging principle of mental health assessment that the ultimate legal opinion is generally not the appropriate focus for the evaluation. Similarly, Melton, Petrila, Poythress, and Slobogin (1997) noted that when forensic practitioners venture to opine on the ultimate issue before the court, they risk overstepping the bounds of competency, even egregiously, by opining about issues outside their areas of expertise or unsupportable by the data. Although there is vigorous debate on this issue within the forensic community, and there is some support for going to the ultimate issue if the data do, indeed, support the opinion, psychologists must give careful consideration to the full range of implications of doing so. Grisso (2003) said, "An expert opinion that answers the ultimate legal question is not an 'expert' opinion, but a personal value judgment" (p. 477).

Psychologists who practice in contexts in which it is expected or required that they answer the legal question may make special effort to temper their opinions, by including cautionary language and caveats regarding the limitations of, and potential influences on, their opinions. The following example may be useful to consider when responding to an ultimate legal question, for example, "How do you think the court should apportion parental responsibility for caregiving for this child?" One might first briefly hesitate to allow time for objection to be offered. Then one might preface the response by making an explicit statement about that being the ultimate issue and therefore the province of the trier of fact, and then couch one's opinion within that limitation, saying something to the effect of,

> Although that question is, of course, a matter for the court to determine, and the court may have a great deal more information than do I to arrive at that determination, I can offer the following observations and opinions, based on the data that I have collected. It is my opinion that . . .

Psychologists may be retained by attorneys or others to answer specific, rather than general, questions. In such instances, psychologists may wonder to what extent they should document potentially related issues that fall outside the question posed. For example, a psychologist may be asked to determine whether a plaintiff has objective memory deficits subsequent to a motor vehicle accident. If the results of the evaluation reveal no cognitive deficits but are consistent with adjustment-related depression, would it be appropriate for the psychologist to simply state that memory was within normal limits, or is the psychologist also responsible for reporting emotional disturbance? The SGFP state, "A full explanation of the results of tests and bases for conclusions should be given" (VII, A2, Public and Professional Communications). The SGFP further state, "Forensic psychologists do not, by either commission or omission, participate in a misrepresentation of their evidence, nor do they participate in partisan attempts to avoid, deny, or subvert the presentation of evidence contrary to their own position" (VII, D). However, the forensic practitioner is also cautioned to report data relevant to the legal question but not to include data extraneous to the question at hand.

Although the psycholegal questions investigated by psychologists and documented in reports may be specifically defined by the client, the psychologist's responsibility in many instances extends beyond the narrow scope of the referral question. For example, some referral sources may not fully appreciate the potential psychological issues involved and thus may not know how to pose the question that they want answered. In addition, the concept of "due diligence" underscores the psychologist's ethical and professional responsibility to address and document substantial medical or psychological problems that were not considered in the referral question (Bush & National Academy of Neuropsychology [NAN] Policy & Planning Committee, 2005):

If failure to document another condition can result in harm to the examinee, the option of nondisclosure may not be ethically viable. If this becomes a point of concern, the neuropsychologist should seek clarification from the retaining party regarding the reason for the limitation posed, present his/her reasoning regarding the presence of a different condition, and consider the judiciousness of accepting cases in which limitations are placed on independence. (p. 1001)

Similarly, even though the court may have narrowly defined a custody evaluation referral—asking the psychologist to evaluate the potential impact of one of the parents' alleged alcohol abuse on the child, for example— the psychologist would nevertheless need to include in reports any other psychopathology or parenting behavior that would likely impact on the child's well-being. This does not mean, however, that the evaluator must report extraneous data that, however interesting or outrageous, has nothing to do with the child's best interest. An example might be the admission, on the part of the litigant, of a transgression that occurred one time, many years before. If the litigant has since demonstrated a clear pattern of acting more appropriately with respect to that behavior or issue, and there is no apparent impact of the earlier behavior on current functioning, it maybe inappropriate to include it in the report. It is, nevertheless, in the evaluator's notes and records, and is discoverable.

Likewise, psychological evaluations conducted in criminal settings often have quite specific referral questions, such as whether the defendant was insane at the time of the alleged offense or competent to waive the Miranda warning and confess at a particular time in the past. Ordinarily, it is prudent to limit the scope of documented opinions regarding such matters to the referral question, as well as the underlying clinical basis for the opinion. However, when referral questions do not address current competency to proceed, and the evaluator has concern about the defendant's ability to understand the nature and consequences of the proceedings and to assist properly in his or her defense, the evaluator has an ethical responsibility to raise the question of the defendant's competency (General Principle A, Beneficence and Nonmaleficence). As this example illustrates, evaluators in the criminal setting have an ethical obligation to safeguard defendants' U.S. Constitutional rights. In this case, the 5th and 14th Amendment rights to due process necessitate a defendant's competency to proceed. Because prosecuting an incompetent defendant violates due-process rights, evaluators must be cognizant of examinee competency and raise the issue when it previously has not been addressed.

The range of issues to be explored and potentially addressed in the report should be anticipated so that the entire range of possibilities can be included when gaining informed consent. The litigant needs to know and have time to consider, for example, that questions may be asked about acting out in adolescence. When there is a sealed record of juvenile adjudication, the litigant may need to have time to consult with counsel regarding rights and responsibilities in responding to the examiner's question. When an issue is irrelevant, because it has no impact on the question before the court, it legitimately can be, and should be, omitted from the report. However, in global assessment of psychological functioning, such as might be requested in a parenting assessment, virtually no issue can be automatically assumed to be irrelevant, and caution is in order when considering whether to omit a finding.

MONITORING SELF-BIAS

The potential for psychologists to sacrifice objectivity in the collection and documentation of information may be particularly prevalent in forensic practice. Failure to consider the possibility of self-bias in forensic practice may represent compromised professional integrity. The SGFP state, "As an expert conducting an evaluation, treatment, consultation, or scholarly–empirical investigation, the forensic psychologist maintains professional integrity by examining the issue at hand from all reasonable perspectives, actively seeking information that will differentially test plausible rival hypotheses" (VI, A2, Methods and Procedures). Psychologists involved in forensic practice must be sensitive to potential sources of bias and guard against the impact of such biases on their work. Although biases may impact data collection and interpretation, their influence tends to become evident in the practitioner's documentation and testimony.

Financial Incentive

The potential for immediate or future financial gain provides considerable incentive for professionals to obtain and present findings that support the position of the retaining party. Although it may be that some attorneys are interested in objective psychological conclusions whether or not their positions are supported, it is certain that a substantial number of attorneys only want to receive psychological reports that unequivocally support their position. Psychologists must guard against threats, however subtle, to their objectivity resulting from financial considerations or from the social pressure to be a part of the "defense team."

Inferential Bias

Coexisting with the potential for financially motivated bias is the susceptibility of psychologists to inferential bias (Deidan & Bush, 2002).

The use of general rules (e.g., heuristics) in the inferential process can result in biases (Faust, 1986) and lead to ethical misconduct. Inferential biases include (a) the availability and representative heuristics, (b) fundamental attribution error, (c) anchoring, (d) confirmatory hypothesis testing, and (e) reconstructive memory. Adverse effects of inferential bias for psychologists include misdiagnosis, inappropriate treatments, exacerbation of symptoms, and inaccurate expert opinions (Darley & Gross, 1983; Sweet & Moulthrop, 1999b). Although these biases may occur in nonforensic psychology practices, the potential for referral sources to repeatedly select practitioners with biases that support their positions may reinforce the bias for the practitioner. Brief descriptions of these five inferential biases follow.

Availability and Representative Heuristics

The *availability heuristic* (Kahneman & Tversky, 1973) occurs when the psychologist attempts to determine the frequency of occurrence of a particular situation, such as a certain diagnosis. Situations stemming from information that is readily available in the psychologist's memory (e.g., frequently encountered diagnoses) are perceived as being more likely to occur, and the psychologist is unlikely to search for less accessible alternative explanations.

The *representative heuristic* (Kahneman & Tversky, 1973) involves categorizing information according to how closely it approximates the characteristics of certain groups. For example, psychologists may classify examinees as "probable malingerers" or "unlikely malingerers" on the basis of their experience with prior examinees with similar symptoms, injuries, or other characteristics.

Fundamental Attribution Error

Fundamental attribution error is the tendency for individuals involved in a situation to overattribute their behaviors to situational requirements and for observers of the same situation to overattribute the individual's behaviors to stable personal characteristics (Ross, 1977). This dynamic makes it more likely for psychologists to attribute patient or examinee symptoms to character traits, whereas patients or examinees will be more likely to attribute their symptoms to external factors.

Susceptibility to this type of error may result from education and training paradigms and from philosophical positions that psychologists may adopt as a result of their experiences. Psychologists make judgments about diagnostic conditions on the basis of their professional experiences and their interpretation of the psychological literature. For example, an expert with considerable experience with traumatic brain injuries may diagnose brain injury when symptoms have psychiatric etiology, whereas a psychologist experienced in evaluating and treating psychotic conditions may infer psychiatric psychogenic etiologies for brain injury sequelae. Some examiners hold extreme positions with regard to certain diagnoses, to the extent that the specific details related to a certain case may have little impact on the opinions rendered. Applying predetermined or formulaic conclusions to individual cases is clearly unethical (Standards 9.06, Interpreting Assessment Results, and 3.01, Unfair Discrimination).

Anchoring

Anchoring involves failure to revise initial impressions, beliefs, or preconceptions despite being faced with new, often contradictory, information. In psychological practice, anchoring may be seen (a) in the formation of preconceptions or opinions from information attained prior to meeting, interviewing, or evaluating a patient or examinee (i.e., prior knowledge) or (b) in the formation of preconceptions or opinions from previous conditions or diagnoses associated with a patient or examinee (i.e., *labeling*; Cantor & Mischel, 1979).

Psychologists' opinions may also be biased by the timing of receipt of information about a patient or examinee, with information obtained first carrying greater weight than information obtained later. Preconceived impressions tend to be durable; once formed, they are difficult to change.

Confirmatory Hypothesis Testing

Pursuing information in such a manner as to influence the information obtained from the person providing the information is known as confirmatory hypothesis testing (Snyder & Campbell, 1980). Psychologists that use a hypothesis-testing approach when gathering background information or administering tests are particularly prone to this type of bias. Although a hypothesis-testing approach allows practitioners to pursue information that they consider to be most relevant to specific referral questions and the unique circumstances of each case, confirmatory hypothesis testing bias may result in psychologists eliciting incomplete or inaccurate information.

Reconstructive Memory

Filling in gaps in memory or altering memory to make it consistent with current experience is known as *reconstructive memory* (Wells, 1982). Although reconstructive memory decreases the likelihood that information will be recalled accurately, people nevertheless tend to be overconfident in their memories and their ability to reconstruct events, conversations, or other important events and information after a period of time has lapsed. This type of bias may be particularly relevant for practice activities that involve evaluation or other psychological services provided for a number of hours across multiple sessions. Delays in completing notes or reports increase the likelihood that some information will be forgotten and later replaced by information that confirms current opinions.

Addressing Self-Bias Proactively

Being aware of the potential for bias in formulating opinions is necessary but not sufficient to avoid falling victim to bias. Taking steps to minimize potential sources of bias and their impact on psychological opinions should be considered an integral component of the forensic evaluation (Brodsky, 1991; Martelli, Bush, & Zasler, 2003). Strategies designed to minimize the potential for bias may involve considering alternative explanations that may disconfirm initial hypotheses (Arkes, 1981; Arnoult & Anderson, 1988), writing explicit arguments for and against proposed opinions (Fischoff, 1982), and generating self-examination questions when formulating opinions (Sweet & Moulthrop, 1999b). To reduce the potential influence of inferential biases, Deidan and Bush (2002) offered multiple recommendations specific to each of the inferential biases discussed earlier.

REPORTS

The written report is the primary vehicle by which the forensic psychologist communicates opinions about the forensic issues of interest that may assist the legal decision maker. Although written reports are not required for all forensic services performed, the vast majority of forensic referrals result in a written report (Melton et al., 1997). Forensic psychological reports tend to differ from clinical reports. Authors of forensic mental health texts describe the elements to be included in forensic reports (e.g., Barsky & Gould, 2002; Heilbrun, 2001; Melton et al., 1997). Minimally, a forensic report includes the purpose of the evaluation, the methods and procedures, the results, and the conclusions. The report should be sufficiently detailed and scientifically based to allow the reader to follow the genesis of the writer's conclusions or opinions (Heilbrun, 2001). Although the report may be the end product of the forensic consultation, it sometimes occurs that testimony, by deposition or in court, is required, and an organized and well-supported report can serve as the foundation for organized, well-supported testimony (Heilbrun, 2001). In contrast, a poorly written report may be used to discredit and embarrass the practitioner (Melton et al., 1997).

The SGFP state,

> Forensic psychologists, by virtue of their competence and rules of discovery, actively disclose all sources of information obtained in the course of their professional services; they actively disclose which information

from which source was used in formulating a particular written product or oral testimony. (VII, E, Public and Professional Communications)

In addition to listing sources of information used, full disclosure would seem to include acknowledging those resources that may have been of value but were unavailable.

Psychologists may be asked to modify reports with regard to format and content. However, any submitted report should be considered final for its purpose (Martelli et al., 2003). When factual errors are found subsequent to the release of the report, the examiner may elect to amend the correct information to the report or revise the original report and state within the revision that it is a corrected version and the rationale for the change. An amendment, rather than a rewriting, may be preferable in that there is less likely to be confusion about the opinion finally being offered, and about how it relates to any earlier opinions offered. The question, "Doctor, just how many reports of yours on this matter are floating around out there?" would be an unpleasant one to face. An amendment, clearly titled as such, is less vulnerable to such criticism.

A request to modify a report that comes from an invested party and reflects that party's self-interest in the outcome of a case represents a request for the psychologist to become a biased advocate, rather than an objective expert (Bush & NAN Policy & Planning Committee, 2005). Such requests should be considered carefully. There are very few acceptable reasons to modify reports once they have been completed, and any modification must ultimately reflect the beliefs of the psychologist rather than those of any other party.

Reproducing Examinee Statements

In criminal evaluation contexts, reproducing defendants' statements in psychological reports has the potential to violate the defendant's due-process rights. This issue arises when evaluating the sanity (mental state at the time of the alleged offense) of a defendant whose competency to proceed has not been established. Evaluating sanity generally requires, among other procedures, interviewing the defendant about the details of the alleged offense to better understand the defendant's intent, motivation, planning, organization, thought process, and general mental status at the time of the offense. Reproducing a defendant's recollected details of a crime can occasionally further the prosecutorial investigation by providing important clues and "leads" that were previously unknown. In essence, the defendant could inadvertently provide a confession that gives the prosecution additional information to follow up on and use against him or her. This issue is addressed in the SGFP:

G. Unless otherwise stipulated by the parties, forensic psychologists are aware that no statements made by a defendant, in the course of any (forensic) examination, no testimony by the expert based on such statements, nor any other fruits of the statements can be admitted into evidence against the defendant in any criminal proceeding, except on an issue respecting mental condition on which the defendant has introduced testimony. Forensic psychologists have an affirmative duty to ensure that their written products and oral testimony conform to this Federal Rule of Procedure (12.2c), or its state equivalent.

1. Because forensic psychologists are often not in a position to know what evidence, documentation, or element of a written product may be or may lend to a "fruit of the statement," they exercise extreme caution in preparing reports or offering testimony prior to the defendant's assertion of a mental state claim or the defendant's introduction of testimony regarding a mental condition. Consistent with the reporting requirements of state or federal law, forensic psychologists avoid including statements from the defendant relating to the time period of the alleged offense.

2. Once a defendant has proceeded to the trial stage, and all pretrial mental health issues such as competency have been resolved, forensic psychologists may include in their reports or testimony any statements made by the defendant that are directly relevant to supporting their expert evidence, providing that the defendant has "introduced" mental state evidence or testimony within the meaning of Federal Rule of Procedure 12.2(c), or its state equivalent. (VI, G1 and G2, Methods and Procedures)

When a defendant's competency to proceed is questionable, his or her competency to waive 5th Amendment rights to silence and avoidance of self-incrimination is also questionable. Ideally, a defendant's competency to proceed should be resolved before addressing sanity; however, it is not uncommon for courts to order mental health evaluations addressing both competency and sanity at the same time. It is generally less of a concern when the evaluation is requested by the defense, depending on work product rules in that particularly jurisdiction (see Melton et al., 1997).

There is little concern when the defendant is clearly competent to decide how much incriminating information he or she wants to provide the evaluator. The issue is also moot when the defendant does not provide incriminating information. However, there are times when either the competency of the defendant is clearly questionable or the information the defendant provides is not only incriminating but also an integral factor in the clinical formulation for a diagnosis or forensic opinion on sanity. In such instances, the psychologist faces a dilemma—whether to provide incriminating information in the report regarding a questionably competent defendant or not being able to explain the rationale for the forensic opinion. Both situations are ethically untenable.

As mentioned, it is simpler to address the competency issue first and have it resolved by the court prior to addressing the sanity issue, but the realities of the criminal setting often do not allow this to occur. One option to resolve this conundrum is to provide a report addressing the defendant's competency and a report addendum addressing the defendant's sanity. The main report contains all the standard clinical information leading to a diagnosis, as well as current mental status and competency to proceed issues. The addendum contains information relating to the investigative details of the offense, the defendant's explanation and description of the offense, and the forensic opinion regarding sanity. This method of reporting works particularly well when responding to court-ordered evaluations because the report and addendum can be sent to the court with a cover letter explaining that because of 5th Amendment issues, the two topics were separated. This information provides the court with the opportunity to release competency-related material first to resolve questions of the defendant's competency. The addendum can then be released to the defense for consideration of a sanity defense and to the prosecution if the defense intends to pursue a sanity defense. In this manner, the court effectively protects the defendant's constitutional rights, and the forensic examiner avoids an ethical conundrum.

Preliminary Reports

It is the practice of some psychologists who perform clinical evaluations and treatment in a forensic context to write a report that is considered, and may be labeled, a *preliminary report*, with the expectation that a "forensic" report may later be requested and produced. Such reports may list the differences between preliminary–clinical and more conclusive–forensic reports in the body of the report. This practice seems to invite the establishment of dual and conflicting roles that occur when transitioning from a clinical examiner to a forensic examiner.

In addition to inviting role conflicts, the use of preliminary reports may be problematic because they are generally offered when not all of the data have been collected, with the caveat that the report will be supplemented when the remaining data are available. The problem with such a practice is that it demonstrates that the evaluator has come to a conclusion of some sort without data that were considered to be important enough to have been sought.

The following sections are taken from a hypothetical "Preliminary Neuropsychological Examination Report":

Introduction section. The purpose of this preliminary neuropsychological evaluation was to examine the patient's neurological functioning from the perspective of her self-reported symptoms, cognitive abilities, behavioral presentation, disability status, and causality. This evaluation is considered preliminary because (a) not all potentially relevant background information has been reviewed; (b) self-reported information has not been corroborated by additional, reliable sources; and (c) alternative explanations for reported and observed difficulties have not been thoroughly considered.

Conclusions section. The results of the evaluation are consistent with a mild traumatic brain injury. The nature and extent of neuropsychological deficits is consistent with a total disability. However, the background information reported by the patient was taken at face value and requires verification by additional sources. . . . This evaluation, despite being preliminary, is considered complete and objective.

The lines from this hypothetical report raise questions of appropriateness for a number of reasons. First, the report is labeled *preliminary*, suggesting that it is being released prematurely, before the necessary information has been obtained and considered. Nevertheless, the report goes on to address forensic issues, such as disability status, in the absence of information that the examiner acknowledges is important. Finally, the examiner makes the misleading statement that there occurred a self-examination of objectivity, despite the existence of statements that are consistent with partiality.

RELEASE OF RAW DATA

The disclosure of raw test data to nonpsychologists, as may be required in forensic practice, presents a unique problem for psychologists (Rapp & Ferber, 2003). The problem involves determining "how to balance the discovery rules, which are designed to provide full disclosure of everything a party will rely on at trial, against the scientific, ethical, and contractual obligations of the psychologist[1] and the test publisher's proprietary interests in the testing instruments" (Rapp & Ferber, 2003, p. 342). For litigation purposes, there is a well-established necessity to disclose the sources of information and methods on which an expert's opinions are based. *FRE 705* states that

The expert may testify in terms of opinion or inference and give reasons therefore without first testifying to the underlying facts or data, unless

---

[1] The term *neuropsychologist* was originally used here but was changed to *psychologist* to reflect the broader application of the quote in this context.

the court requires otherwise. The expert may in any event be required to disclose the underlying facts or data on cross-examination. (*FRE*, 1993)

In contrast to the benefits of disclosure in litigation, far-reaching negative consequences may flow from wide dissemination of psychological evaluation methods and procedures. As a result, psychologists working in forensic contexts may struggle with how to negotiate the competing demands of the legal system and their profession.

The 2002 APA Ethics Code represents a significant departure from the 1992 Ethics Code (APA, 1992) and from other sources of ethical authority on the matter of release of test data. In the 1992 Ethics Code, psychologists were instructed to "make reasonable efforts to maintain the integrity and security of tests and other assessment techniques consistent with law, contractual obligations, and in a manner that permits compliance with this code" (Standard 2.10, Maintaining Test Security). In contrast, the 2002 Ethics Code distinguished *test materials* from *test data*. "*Test materials* refers to manuals, instruments, protocols, and test questions or stimuli" (Standard 9.11, Maintaining Test Security). *Test materials* do not include test data: "Psychologists make reasonable efforts to maintain the integrity and security of test materials and other assessment techniques consistent with law and contractual obligations, and in a manner that permits adherence to this Ethics Code" (Standard 9.11). Thus, the Ethics Code speaks to the importance of safeguarding psychological tests to avoid potential damage that would result to the profession and potential clients if such measures were made available to those who were not qualified to use them.

In contrast to *test materials*, Standard 9.04a, Release of Test Data, defines *test data* as "raw and scaled scores, client/patient responses to test questions or stimuli, and psychologists' notes and recordings concerning client/patient statements and behavior during an examination." To address the problem of physically separating the test data from the test materials, Standard 9.04a states, "Those portions of test materials that include client/patient responses are included in the definition of *test data*." Clarification from the APA Ethics Office indicated that once test materials have responses written on them, they "convert" to test data (Behnke, 2003). This position suggests that test materials, which enjoy protection under Standard 9.11, Maintaining Test Security, are no longer test materials and no longer enjoy such protection once they have answers written on them. This same premise apparently applies to test materials that are reproduced by examinees as their responses, such as verbal learning tests and visual reproduction tests.

Standard 9.04a, Release of Test Data, states, "Pursuant to a client/patient release, psychologists provide test data to the client/patient or other persons identified in the release." That is, according to the APA Ethics Code, psychologists are to provide test data to anyone whom the client or patient specifies. In many forensic contexts, the attorney or court may determine to whom the data are released. Standard 9.04a does offer exceptions to the obligatory release at the behest of the client or patient:

> Psychologists may refrain from releasing test data to protect a client/ patient or others from substantial harm or misuse or misinterpretation of the data or the test, recognizing that in many instances release of confidential information under these circumstances is regulated by law.

Celia B. Fisher (2003b), PhD, Chair of the APA's Ethics Code Task Force, defined *substantial harm* as "reasonably likely to endanger the life or physical safety of the individual or another person or cause equally substantial harm" (p. 12). Forensic psychologists working with death penalty cases may represent an exception to this standard. Psychologists in such situations would likely not be able to defend withholding test data on the grounds that releasing the data could result in the application of the substantial harm of the death penalty to the examinee.

The misinterpretation or misuse clause may pose greater challenges for psychologists. Psychologists may wonder, "How could data not be misinterpreted or misused in the hands of those not trained to interpret them?" They may further wonder, "How could misinterpretation or misuse not be harmful?" When psychologists have undergone years of education and training to be competent to interpret psychological tests, they may find it unlikely that people who lack such training could interpret those tests appropriately. Rapp and Ferber (2003) noted that "the client's test answers, with the psychologist's analysis, are meaningless to, and likely to be misinterpreted by, anyone other than a specifically trained psychologist" (p. 353). However, C. B. Fisher (2003b) cautioned, "Before refusing to release test data under this clause, psychologists should carefully review relevant law. HIPAA (Health Insurance Portability and Accountability Act; U.S. Department of Health and Human Services [U.S. DHHS], 1996) does not recognize the protection of test materials as a legitimate reason to withhold designated record sets appropriately requested by a client/patient" (p. 12).

C. B. Fisher (2003b) also indicated that "The extent to which HIPAA, state privacy rules, and Standard 9.04 of the Ethics Code will conflict with test copyright laws will be determined over time" (p. 12). Such clarification has been provided by Richard Campanelli, Director of the Office for Civil Rights at the U.S. DHHS, the office responsible for the administration of the 1996 HIPAA. Campanelli stated,

> Any requirement for disclosure of protected health information pursuant to the Privacy Rule is subject to Section 1172(e) of HIPAA, "Protection of Trade Secrets." As such, we confirm that it would not be a violation of the Privacy Rule for a covered entity to refrain from providing access to an individual's protected health information, to the extent that

doing so would result in a disclosure of trade secrets. (Multi-Health Systems, 2003)

Thus, HIPAA does not prohibit psychologists from withholding test data when the potential for misinterpretation or misuse exists, and such action may be a viable option in some situations.

In forensic evaluation contexts, some HIPAA constraints are not relevant (Connell & Koocher, 2003; C. B. Fisher, 2003b). HIPAA states that information compiled in anticipation of use in civil, criminal, and administrative proceedings is not subject to the same right of review and amendment as is health care information in general (§164.524(a)(1)(ii); U.S. DHHS, 1996). Although HIPAA may not fully apply to forensic evaluation cases, other relevant laws do apply.

The APA Ethics Code (Standard 9.04b, Release of Test Data) permits psychologists to release data, without client–patient consent, in response to a court order or other legal authority (C. B. Fisher, 2003b). However, psychologists need not automatically release data in such situations without taking steps to safeguard test materials. C. B. Fisher (2003b) stated, "Psychologists may ask the court or other legal authority for a protective order to prevent the inappropriate disclosure of confidential information or suggest that the information be submitted to another psychologist for qualified review" (p. 12). The importance of maximizing test security in the context of requests for test data or materials has been emphasized by the NAN Policy & Planning Committee (2000b, 2005), and specific steps to safeguard test materials have been outlined.

Psychologists should avail themselves of additional sources of ethical and legal authority that address this issue. The SGFP (VII, A2a and A2b, Public and Professional Communications) and the Standards for Educational and Psychological Testing (SEPT; Standards 11.7, 11.8, and 11.9; American Educational Research Association, APA, & National Council on Measurement in Education, 1999) acknowledge the importance of maintaining test security and ensuring that only those qualified to interpret raw test scores be afforded access to do so. Standard 11.7 of the SEPT states that

> Test users have the responsibility to protect the security of tests, to the extent that developers enjoin users to do so. . . . When tests are involved in litigation, inspection of the instruments should be restricted—to the extent permitted by law—to those who are legally or ethically obligated to safeguard test security. (p. 115)

SEPT Standard 11.8 states, "Test users have the responsibility to respect test copyrights" (p. 115). When purchasing psychological tests, psychologists agree to uphold copyright laws. In SEPT Standard 11.15, the potential for misinterpretation of test data is addressed: "Test users should be alert to potential misinterpretations of test scores and to possible unintended consequences of test use; users should take steps to minimize or avoid foreseeable misinterpretations and unintended negative consequences" (p. 116).

Jurisdictional laws regarding patients' rights to access their medical records must also be considered. Such laws may conflict with ethical demands. When conflicts between legal and ethical requirements exist, psychologists are obligated to try to find ways to meet the requirements of both (Standard 1.02, Conflicts Between Ethics and Law, Regulations, or Other Governing Legal Authority). In cases in which no solution adequately satisfies both demands, psychologists "ultimately must let their own personal conscience guide them" (Slick & Iverson, 2003, p. 2032).

These two potential courses of action (releasing or safeguarding raw test data) pit fundamental ethical principles against each other. Providing data to the client is consistent with respecting the right of the client to choose what is done with the work product for which they contracted (autonomy; General Principle E, Respect for People's Rights and Dignity). In contrast, providing data to an individual who is not qualified to interpret them and is not bound by the same ethical requirement to safeguard them may result in harm to the examinee (General Principle A, Beneficence and Nonmaleficence) and may result in invalidation of future examinations of others (General Principle D, Justice). In dilemmas such as this, the greater harm must be determined. Disservice to many would likely outweigh the restricted service to one. However, as Rapp and Ferber (2003) stated, "The harm from disclosure can be avoided while still accommodating the opposing side's legitimate need to prepare its case" (p. 352). Access to raw test data and materials can be limited to psychologists, or a protective order can be obtained, to maximize test security and minimize the potential for harm, and still conform to discovery rules. In addition to conflicting ethical principles, however, relevant legal authorities may conflict, and the psychologist may be required by law to release raw test data to individuals not properly trained to interpret them. In those circumstances, the psychologist makes known the relevant concerns, in writing or "on the record," and then follows the directive of the law (APA Ethics Code, Introduction and Applicability).

The importance of maintaining test security and avoiding misuse, misinterpretation, or other potentially harmful uses of test data is clearly recognized by sources of ethical authority. However, integrating these concerns with the right to disclosure that is attendant to most court proceedings may be challenging in some contexts. It appears that solely on the basis of the APA Ethics Code, psychologists could, with client release if needed, justify immediately releasing test data (including test materials on which responses have been written) to anyone identified by the client, or alternatively, could justify taking steps to safeguard the test data and materials. Because either course of action may be supported by the Ethics Code, psychologists must decide for themselves whether they want to do what is simply ethically acceptable (i.e., release the data) or what may be considered ethically preferable (i.e., take steps to limit access to the data and materials; Bush, 2004a). Consultation with one's own attorney may be advisable.

Although Standard 9.04, Release of Test Data, apparently represents an effort to make the APA Ethics Code more consistent with the anticipated implications of HIPAA (C. B. Fisher, 2003b), HIPAA makes no demand that psychologists release trade secrets in the form of test materials or data. Thus, the dramatic change in Standard 9.04 does not seem to have met the goal for which it was intended. Instead, Standard 9.04 has served to conflict with the other relevant section of the Ethics Code (Standard 9.11, Maintaining Test Security), with general bioethical principles, and with other sources of ethical authority, and it has caused confusion for psychologists. Psychologists releasing raw test data to those not qualified to interpret them, in the absence of a court order, should carefully consider their motivations for departing from the majority of sources of ethical authority. Psychologists should carefully consider the available options that might allow them to achieve conformity with their own and authoritative concepts of ethical practice.

Clinicians Thwarting Disclosure

In their desire to protect their patients, some clinicians may attempt to prevent disclosure of their records (Barsky & Gould, 2002). The following strategies may be used to thwart disclosure: keeping minimal records, keeping double sets of records, coding information in their records, doctoring or disposing of records and documents, or outright lying (Barsky & Gould, 2002). Each of these actions, although motivated by a desire to protect or help the patient, represents ethical misconduct, with the exception that psychotherapy notes may indeed be maintained as a separate set of records. *Psychotherapy notes*, as defined by HIPAA, may be kept separate from other client records and may not be easily obtainable. HIPAA (§164.501; U.S. DHHS, 1996) defined such notes:

> Psychotherapy notes means notes recorded (in any medium) by a health care provider who is a mental health professional documenting or analyzing the contents of conversation during a private counseling session or a group, joint, or family counseling session and that are separated from the rest of the individual's medical record. Psychotherapy notes excludes medication prescription and monitoring, counseling session start and stop times, the modalities and frequencies of treatment furnished, results of clinical tests, and any summary of the following items: diagnosis, functional status, the treatment plan, symptoms, prognosis, and progress to date.

Thus, without the explicit consent of the therapy patient, the therapist may not be able to release psychotherapy notes, and to be defined as such, those notes must have been kept separate from the rest of the patient's file. In this one regard, the maintenance of two sets of records is, of course, not unethical at all, and refusal to disclose the psychotherapy notes is not objectionable. In cases involving court-ordered treatment, there is less clarity in HIPAA regarding the protection of such notes, and arguably, given that the treatment is occurring in a litigation context, there may be little protection of the records.

Maintaining records sufficient to serve the clinical or forensic purposes of the treatment or evaluation may be the best way to avoid ethical misconduct. Practitioners in many contexts should anticipate that requests for the records will be made, and they should maintain documentation accordingly.

FEEDBACK

Psychologists in clinical settings should typically share test results and interpretations with the test taker; however, judicial referrals represent one exception to the ethical and professional requirement to provide feedback (Standard 9.10, Explaining Assessment Results; SEPT, Standard 12.20). In the context of examinations by psychological experts retained by opposing counsel (e.g., independent medical examinations), psychologists typically do not provide examinees with feedback regarding results, conclusions, or recommendations. Reports are released to the retaining party, not to examinees or their family members, doctors, lawyers, or other representatives without the permission of the retaining party (Bush & NAN Policy & Planning Committee, 2005). Similarly, in court-ordered child custody evaluations, the evaluator may elect to release the report to the court and the attorneys, without giving feedback directly to the parties, and in fact, it is not unusual for the court to direct the manner in which the evaluator's findings will be released. HIPAA does not seem to protect the examinee's right to access and amend psychological records in forensic contexts (Connell & Koocher, 2003; U.S. DHHS, 1996). The examinee should understand the extent and nature of the feedback that will be provided, if any, and to whom it will be provided, before the evaluation is begun.

CASE 4: ANTICIPATING INVOLVEMENT IN
A PERSONAL INJURY CASE

A single 35-year-old accountant sustains a severe brain injury when thrown from his horse while riding on his own property. He recovers well.

Although he is able to live independently, persisting cognitive deficits prohibit his return to work. Emotional distress emerges. He begins treatment with a psychologist during inpatient rehabilitation and continues psychotherapy on an outpatient basis in her private practice, paying out of pocket. Treatment covers the patient's accident-related changes as well as longstanding, sensitive family problems. A caring therapeutic relationship develops. The psychologist keeps detailed notes of the therapy and has test results from early in treatment. A few months into treatment, the patient mentions that his family is considering a lawsuit against the hospital, although he is unsure of the details. Within a week, the psychologist receives a request for her records, accompanied by a signed consent to release, from the attorney representing her patient. She goes back through her progress notes and finds very sensitive and personal information. She briefly considers what to do.

Analysis

Identify the Problem

The psychologist did not want to release sensitive patient information. She did not have a strong opinion about releasing raw test data and did not see this as a sensitive issue.

Consider the Significance of the Context and Setting

The psychologist was treating the patient in her independent practice, with no institutional support and little collegial support. Similar requests that came to the rehabilitation hospital were handled by the medical records and legal departments, and she was almost never involved. She was unprepared for a situation that would inevitably arise in a rehabilitation-related practice.

Identify and Use Ethical and Legal Resources

A number of ethical, professional, and legal resources were available to the psychologist. A review of these resources, had it occurred, would have revealed the following. Her desire to protect her patient was consistent with General Principle A (Beneficence). Due primarily to a lack of experience in this treatment context, she was unaware of potential courses of action that would best serve her patient, herself, the profession of psychology, and the legal system (Standard 2.01, Boundaries of Competence). Altering and destroying records would violate Standard 6.01, Documentation of Professional Work and Maintenance of Records, and producing notes with new and potentially different content would be inconsistent with Standard 5.01, Avoidance of False or Deceptive Statements, and with the law. The psychologist's state laws prohibited destruction of medical records.

Releasing raw test data without taking steps to safeguard them would be inappropriate, according to some sources of ethical authority (NAN Policy & Planning Committee, 2000b, 2005; SEPT Standards 11.7, 11.8, and 11.9). The General Principle D (Justice) could be considered applicable to both sides of this issue. Releasing the data would serve the justice system, as well as help her patient's case (Beneficence). However, the potentially adverse consequences of uncontrolled dissemination could include invalidation of the tests, which could potentially deny future examinees their right to access and benefit from the contributions of psychology, thus potentially harming the public. Further, test developers and publishers who may have spent great effort and cost to bring the tests to market, and who have copyrights, would be damaged by uncontrolled distribution and resultant invalidation of the instruments. Such damage to test developers and publishers would have repercussions for psychological practice. When conflicts exist between or within principles, a determination or judgment regarding the potential for the greatest harm and the greatest benefit must be made. The psychologist's state laws were consistent with the release of all records with the patient's consent.

Failing to discuss the potential therapeutic and personal implications of releasing sensitive information with her patient would reflect a lack of appreciation of the importance of individual autonomy (General Principle E, Respect for People's Rights and Dignity).

Consider Personal Beliefs and Values

The psychologist's primary motivation was the wish to help her patient. She believed that protecting her patient would justify almost any behavior she chose, including the destruction and modification of records. She had never given much thought to the issues surrounding release of data. She was aware that, with signed consent from the patient, the APA Ethics Code allowed her to release her records, and she gave the issue no further thought.

Develop Possible Solutions to the Problem

The psychologist briefly considered releasing her current record as it was. She then considered revising her progress notes to eliminate the sensitive personal information that the patient had shared and to focus on accident-related content. She considered making up details to fill in notes in which session content was uncertain or scantily recorded. She briefly considered calling a colleague but could not think of anyone to call. She also considered posting her dilemma on a professional electronic discussion board and asking for advice. She did not consider contacting the ethics committee of a professional organization; taking time to weigh the potential advantages and consequences of various courses of action, making notes of the issues being weighed; or discussing the issues with her patient.

Choose and Implement a Course of Action

The psychologist rewrote some of her notes, shredding the originals. She then copied and sent to the court the remaining entire record, including the revised notes, test reports, and test data. The psychologist acted without giving much thought, if any, to other possible courses of action. She opted to do what she considered to be in the patient's best interest, without regard for the potential ethical and legal implication.

Assess the Outcome and Implement Changes as Needed

No one ever knew that the psychologist modified and destroyed records. The release of raw test data was supported by her state laws and the APA Ethics Code and, therefore, created no problems. The violation of copyright laws was never alleged. Treatment continued as it had before, although the psychologist anticipated that subsequent notes would be subject to review by others and thus omitted detailed sensitive information. On the basis of her experience with this patient, she modified her informed consent and note-writing procedures to avoid such problems in the future.

Comment

Although not necessarily unethical according to the APA Ethics Code, the psychologist's release of raw test data without taking steps to safeguard them, and her failure to uphold her copyright obligation, may be construed to be marginally acceptable practice. She failed to consult with a knowledgeable colleague when she found herself in an unfamiliar and uncomfortable situation. She failed to discuss the potential implications of releasing the records with her patient, who may have chosen to rescind his consent. Had the psychologist thought through, either by herself or with a colleague, the potential ethical and legal implications of her options before acting, she would have been in a better position to serve her patient, herself, and the profession of psychology.

6

TESTIMONY AND TERMINATION

The psychologist's activities in a forensic matter may change as the status of the case changes, progresses, and nears conclusion. Care must be taken at case transition points to ensure that (a) services already provided do not conflict with or contaminate anticipated activities and (b) future activities do not undermine services previously provided. Testimony and termination are transition points at which psychologists may be well served by clarifying prior understandings with the retaining party, reaffirming a commitment to accuracy, understanding attorney tactics, and anticipating responsibilities associated with the conclusion of the case. This chapter reviews ethical and professional considerations related to roles, accuracy, attorney tactics, and maintenance and disclosure of records in the context of testimony and termination.

ROLE CLARIFICATION

Clarification of the roles that psychologists and clients establish at the outset of professional interactions may be necessary at multiple points during the provision of psychological services. The transition from treatment or evaluation to testimony is one point at which role clarification may be particularly important. Forensic testimony often provides enticement or unintended opportunity for psychologists to engage in two or more roles

113

with a single client, patient, or examinee. Some attorneys and courts have a preference for treating psychologists (vs. independent experts) to provide expert testimony regarding forensic issues and may instruct or entice psychologists to blur role boundaries or to engage in clear dual roles. When asked or required to testify, practitioners should assess the potential for deviation from the role agreed upon at the outset of service provision. When considering adopting dual or multiple roles, psychologists should carefully consider the potential for reduced objectivity and effectiveness and for exploitation or harm to the patient or examinee (Heilbrun, 2001).

Treating psychologists must be aware that offering testimony about forensic issues is risky for three primary reasons. First, in treatment contexts, the nature and extent of the background and evaluation data obtained may be insufficient, and the manner in which they were obtained may lack the skepticism required for critical review (S. Greenberg & Shuman, 1997). Second, the existence of an established treatment relationship may reduce the impartiality that is typically required for unbiased testimony regarding forensic issues. Treating psychologists tend to be appropriately empathic, wanting the best for their patients. However, this stance is inconsistent with impartiality (S. Greenberg & Shuman, 1997). Third, and perhaps most important, the assumption of the role of forensic evaluator or testifying expert may interfere with the patient's treatment. For these reasons, the need to generally avoid potentially harmful dual or multiple relationships is an established principle (American Academy of Psychiatry and the Law, 1995; American Psychological Association [APA], 2002; Committee on Ethical Guidelines for Forensic Psychologists, 1991; S. Greenberg & Shuman, 1997; Heilbrun, 2001) and should be considered when asked to testify.

The need to inform the examinee, in a manner that can be understood, of the nature of the psychologist–examinee relationship is fundamental to the informed consent and notification of purpose process. Deviations from the initial mutually agreed upon relationship should generally be avoided. Psychologists are advised to be vigilant to attorneys' efforts, throughout the provision of psychological services, to induce them to take on multiple roles; for example, there may be tendencies for attorneys to ask questions during testimony that would require the psychologist to cross role boundaries.

ACCURACY

Expert testimony is an integral component of forensic psychological services, even though it is required in only a minority of cases (Heilbrun, 2001). Testimony, as an extension of the written report, should be based on the integration of relevant research and the information gathered in the conduct of the evaluation. Anchoring conclusions to the data reduces the potential for bias to sway the evaluator when articulating opinions in reports and testimony (Heilbrun, 2001).

Effective expert testimony requires attention to both style and substance of presentation (Heilbrun, 2001). Effectiveness in style alone, or in substance without style, considerably limits the psychologist's contribution to the court. Although a communication style that resonates with the trier of fact adds considerably to the value of the expert's testimony, psychological ethics traditionally focus solely on the accuracy, rather than style, of communication. Standard 5.01, Avoidance of False or Deceptive Statements, of the APA Ethics Code (2002) states, "Psychologists do not knowingly make public statements that are false, deceptive, or fraudulent." The Ethics Code also requires psychologists to base the opinions expressed in their reports and forensic testimony on information and techniques sufficient to substantiate their findings (Standards 2.04, Bases for Scientific and Professional Judgments, and 9.01, Bases for Assessments). In addition, the Specialty Guidelines for Forensic Psychologists (SGFP; VII, D, Public and Professional Communications; Committee on Ethical Guidelines for Forensic Psychologists, 1991) note that when testifying, psychologists should not, either actively or passively, engage in partisan distortion or misrepresentation.

ATTORNEY TACTICS

Attorneys may attempt to elicit false testimony from the expert on the stand. In such instances, it may be beneficial to pause before answering, thus allowing the retaining attorney an opportunity to object. If such objection is not forthcoming, the psychologist should restate the correct opinion, as forcefully as is necessary. The SGFP (VII, D, Public and Professional Communications) state that forceful representation of the data and reasoning on which one's opinion is based is not precluded, as long as the information is presented accurately.

Attorneys may inaccurately represent an expert's opinion. When psychologists become aware of such attempts, it is necessary to correct the misinformation. Standard 1.01, Misuse of Psychologists' Work, states, "If psychologists learn of misuse or misrepresentation of their work, they take reasonable steps to correct or minimize the misuse or misrepresentation." In addition, the SGFP (VII, D, Public and Professional Communications) state, "Forensic psychologists do not, by either commission or omission, participate in a misrepresentation of their evidence, nor do they participate in partisan attempts to avoid, deny, or subvert the presentation of evidence contrary to their own position."

COMPLETION OF THE CASE

The relationship between the forensic psychologist and the retaining party, in a specific case, typically ends when the report has been submitted, testimony has been provided, or payment for services has been received (Bush & National Academy of Neuropsychology [NAN] Policy & Planning Committee, 2005). As part of the contract for services established at the outset of the relationship, the psychologist and the retaining party should agree on the point at which the case will be considered completed. The psychologist's willingness to respond to subsequent requests for reports or data may be determined by the status of the relationship with the retaining party. Similarly, the psychologist should establish in advance who will hold the privilege (who is responsible for protecting the examinee's confidentiality) regarding the psychological data and results following termination of the relationship.

In some cases, an examinee may request treatment from the psychologist after the conclusion of the case. S. Greenberg and Shuman (1997) noted that ethical concerns exist in "the subsequent provision of therapy by a psychologist or psychiatrist who previously provided a forensic assessment of that litigant" (p. 50). The contrasting position is that if the examination relationship has ended and the forensic action that initiated the examination has been completed, the psychologist may consider providing such treatment. However, the psychologist who, as the former forensic examiner, elects to subsequently provide therapy must be prepared to defend the decision to not refer the examinee to another qualified professional. The primary concern is for the welfare of the potential patient.

A notable exception is any case involving the best interest of a child. The evaluator's role as impartial expert to the court continues, in a sense, until the child reaches majority, and to take on any treatment relationship with a party to the matter may deprive one of the parties or the court of the advantage to be gained by further access to the impartial and objective opinion of the expert who was originally court appointed or who did an evaluation by agreement of the parties. The professional guidelines for custody evaluation promulgated by the APA (1994) state, "Therapeutic contact with the child or involved participants following a child custody evaluation is undertaken with caution"; absent compelling circumstances, such treatment seems ill-advised.

There may be treatment-related reasons to avoid assuming this secondary role, a principle reason being that the more investigative and less empathically resonant posture of the examiner is quite different from that of the treating clinician, and may thus lay a predicate for a nontherapeutic environment (S. Greenberg & Shuman, 1997). Finally, the forensic evaluator who stands to gain financially from recommending ongoing treatment is vulnerable to compromised objectivity when considering such a recommendation. A recommendation that the examinee return to the forensic examiner for therapy would typically represent a conflict of interest. In practice, then, it is almost always ill-advised to accept this second role. Nevertheless, in situations in which it is deemed appropriate to assume a second role as a therapist, once the treating relationship has been established, further independent examinations would be prohibited (Bush & NAN Policy & Planning Committee, 2005).

MAINTENANCE OF RECORDS

Psychologists are required to maintain records of cases in which they have testified and to provide that information when appropriate requests are made (Standards 6.01, Documentation of Professional and Scientific Work and Maintenance of Records, and 6.02, Maintenance, Dissemination, and Disposal of Confidential Records of Professional and Scientific Work). Because examinees, or their legal representatives, have made their psychological status a matter of legal scrutiny, relevant information may fall in the public domain. As a result, confidentiality concerns should be carefully considered and the information provided to authorized parties in a methodical, well-documented fashion.

CASE 5: DISCLOSURE OF TEST RESULTS IN CRIMINAL CASES

A forensic psychologist receives a referral from a criminal defense attorney to evaluate her client regarding competency to stand trial. This is his first referral from this attorney. The defendant, it is alleged, received multiple blows to the body and head at the time of his arrest 3 months prior and is now suffering from severe posttraumatic stress disorder (PTSD), rendering him incompetent to stand trial. The psychologist performs an appropriately complete evaluation that includes a personality inventory and a separate measure of symptom validity. Evaluation results reveal considerable emotional distress; however, symptom validity indicators are variable. Scores on the validity scales of the personality inventory are within normal limits. In contrast, performance on the symptom validity test (SVT) reflects a tendency to endorse numerous symptoms in an indiscriminant manner, consistent with symptom fabrication or exaggeration. The evaluator concludes that the defendant's performance on the SVT can be explained by legitimate emotional distress. He provides a verbal account of his findings to the defense attorney, reporting that he believes the defendant to be not competent to stand trial because of severe PTSD. At the request of defense counsel, he then writes a report outlining the evaluation results and opinion.

During preparation for testimony, the attorney requests the psychologist recount results of the clinical tests but not "muddy the waters" by discussing the SVT results, because the interpretation of the personality inventory results, as reported, is that they are the result of emotional distress and not malingering. The psychologist is concerned about presenting only a portion of the results, but the attorney seems strongly committed to providing only information that "facilitates the defense strategy." The psychologist wants to do a good job with this case to generate more referrals from this attorney in the future.

Analysis

Identify the Problem

The psychologist was instructed by the attorney to not discuss, during testimony, aspects of the test results that might reflect negatively on the criminal defendant because it would not facilitate the defense strategy. The expert agreed with the attorney's representation of the basic thrust of his opinions as they were to be communicated through testimony, but he felt uncomfortable not outlining potentially contradictory test results and explaining them. He was faced with a dilemma regarding withholding data, on the basis that they were irrelevant and that offering them would simply confuse the trier of fact, when in fact such withholding was being requested to advance defense aims. He certainly did not wish to unnecessarily muddy the waters.

Consider the Significance of the Context and Setting

The legal setting demands that mental health experts answer questions posed by attorneys. Experts do not control the nature of the questions, and there is considerable variability in the amount of off-topic responding an expert can do. In this instance, the evaluator knew beforehand that the attorney intended to draw forth testimony about the personality inventory, while avoiding testimony about the SVT. When prepared regarding the question, "Doctor, please tell the court about the manner in which you determined the test results were valid," the expert was asked to present only a portion of the information. Even though testimony is structured by attorney questions, the law requires the witness to tell the "the truth, whole truth, and nothing but the truth." The psychologist was also concerned about doing the right thing for the defendant; he did not want to unnecessarily harm the defendant. He was also concerned about his professional relationship with the defense attorney; he was hopeful that he might receive additional cases from this referral source.

Identify and Use Ethical and Legal Resources

The psychologist, in his deliberations about the dilemma, considered biomedical ethical principles and referred to the APA Ethics Code, the SGFP, and relevant texts. The psychologist considered the principle of nonmaleficence but had some difficulty discerning which parties would be harmed if he testified either in full or in part. Testifying fully about the invalid SVT results would harm the defendant's case; however, the psychologist considered that his primary obligation was to the truth, not to the defendant or to the defense attorney. Failure to acknowledge the SVT results would be harmful to the justice system, and potentially to society, and would be inconsistent with the principle of justice.

The APA Ethics Code (Standard 5.01, Avoidance of False or Deceptive Statements) instructs psychologists to avoid false or deceptive statements, including statements in legal proceedings. Failure to testify about test data that potentially contradict his opinions would be deceptive. In addition, psychologists must describe any significant limitations of test data interpretation (Standard 9.06, Interpreting Assessment Results); the examinee's performance on the SVT posed a clear limitation on his interpretation that should have been addressed in reports or testimony.

The SGFP reveal that

> forensic psychologists make reasonable efforts to ensure that the products of their services, as well as their own public statements and professional testimony, are communicated in ways that will promote understanding and avoid deception, given the particular characteristics, roles, and abilities of various recipients of the communications. (VII, A, Public and Professional Communications)

Further, the SGFP point out that "forensic psychologists take reasonable steps to correct misuse or misrepresentation of their professional products, evidence, and testimony," (VII, A1) and that "a full explanation of the results of tests and the bases for conclusions should be given in language that the client can understand" (VII, A2). Last, the SGFP indicate that

> When testifying, forensic psychologists have an obligation to all parties to a legal proceeding to present their findings, conclusions, evidence, or other professional products in a fair manner . . . Forensic psychologists do not, by either commission or omission, participate in a misrepresentation of their evidence, nor do they participate in partisan attempts to avoid, deny, or subvert the presentation of evidence contrary to their own position. (VII, D)

In his review of professional literature, the psychologist found a consistent theme reflecting the ethical obligation of psychologists to fully disclose the nature of their findings (Grisso, 2003; Heilbrun, 2001). The psychologist interpreted "fully disclose" to include those evaluation findings that were potentially contradictory to the conclusions reached but were ultimately dismissed or were accounted for in a manner that was consistent with the conclusions reached.

Consider Personal Beliefs and Values

The psychologist takes seriously his legal mandate to "tell the whole truth, and nothing but the truth" during testimony. He believes that just as it is not helpful to leave out important and relevant aspects of the data, it is also not helpful to discuss a laundry list of marginally relevant points. In this instance the psychologist was faced not only with external pressure from the attorney but also with internal pressures to serve this referral source well and to avoid doing something that might unnecessarily harm the defendant's case.

Develop Possible Solutions to the Problem

The psychologist was aware of his unease about limiting his testimony and addressing only the favorable validity test. First, he considered complying with the attorney's request under the reasoning that this was a legal case, the attorney's case at that, so he should just do what she said and not worry about it. To do so, however, he would have to ignore his discomfiture and worry that he was not telling the "whole truth." Second, he considered the option of agreeing to this plan with the attorney but testifying in a forthcoming way when asked about validity issues. He realized this broadsiding of the attorney would be dishonest as well. He wanted to balance doing the right thing with being forthright and reasonable. Third, he considered openly addressing his concerns with the defense attorney prior to testifying. He considered that an honest conversation with the attorney about these issues may reveal that the attorney did not want him to misrepresent his findings or opinion and that she was probably so focused on defense strategy that she was not thinking through the issues. By following this course of action and standing up for his own principles, he could actually increase the attorney's respect for him.

Choose and Implement a Course of Action

The psychologist determined he simply could not omit the SVT results from his testimony. He could also not mislead the attorney by agreeing to do so and then doing the opposite when testifying. He decided it was more professionally appropriate to demonstrate respect for the attorney and her client by being forthright and direct about the matter. He respected her expertise but also knew that her professional mandate—to provide zealous representation—was not the mandate under which he must practice. He needed to follow his own conscience, the rules of testimony, and his ethical obligations as he understood them. He told the attorney it was inappropriate for him to omit the SVT results and recommended they take the time during testimony to explain the importance of using multiple measures of response validity and integrating the test results and clinical findings in their entirety. He pointed out that including and explaining even potentially negative results would advance his own credibility as a responsible expert. He also expressed his conviction that he would not be testifying to the whole truth if he did not explain these potentially negative test results.

Assess the Outcome and Implement Changes as Needed

After some hesitancy, the defense attorney agreed that full disclosure could potentially increase the psychologist's credibility and that they could take the time, in testimony, to carefully explain the results. She conceded she did not want him betray his obligation to tell the truth. When he testified and explained the results in their entirety, the testimony went well. After the hearing, the attorney voiced her appreciation for his professionalism and agreed that by explaining even potentially negative aspects of the results, the principle points of his testimony were made stronger. She said she hoped to share other cases with him in the future.

7

ADDRESSING ETHICAL MISCONDUCT

As the previous chapters illustrate, there are many factors that can contribute to ethically questionable conduct or clear misconduct on the part of psychologists. Some ethical misconduct is intentional, and some is unintentional.

Forensic practice exposes psychologists' work to greater scrutiny than is typical in other areas of practice. Such critical review by colleagues can lead to strong defensive reactions, sometimes justified and sometimes not. In addition, the conclusions reached by psychologists are likely to be based on multiple sources of data, some of which are inconsistent (Heilbrun, 2001). The inconsistent aspects of the data, if not appropriately addressed by the examiner, can become a source of contention between the examiner and an independent reviewer. As Heilbrun noted, "There are sometimes reasonable alternative explanations or conclusions that would be possible within the context of a single case" (p. 227). Disagreement regarding potential explanations or conclusions can become points of contention, particularly among psychologists who are strongly wedded to a certain perspective regarding the condition being considered. Psychologists are often powerful and persuasive advocates of their positions, and they may sometimes stretch the boundaries of appropriate or justified testimony to make poorly supported statements, or engage in behavior, to advance their positions.

Financial incentive can also contribute to ethical misconduct. Compared with psychological practice in many health care settings, forensic practice offers the potential for substantially greater income. In clinical settings, income typically is not tied directly or indirectly to the findings of competent examinations. Motivation for increased income may motivate some psychologists practicing in forensic settings to engage in practices that they might not consider in clinical settings. In addition, the adversarial nature of forensic practice may result in strong and, at times, personal feelings toward psychologists retained by the opposing side. Such feelings may, appropriately or inappropriately, bias one's perspective of the work of those colleagues.

Theses factors, as well as other aspects of forensic practice, may contribute to psychologists perceiving the work of colleagues as unethical. When psychologists perceive the behavior of a colleague to be unethical and consider possible courses of action, they are advised to examine various factors that may influence their decisions. The following framework for addressing perceived ethical misconduct by colleagues is offered as a means of organizing psychologists' decision making in this context.

FRAMEWORK FOR ADDRESSING PERCEIVED ETHICAL MISCONDUCT

Determining an appropriate response to perceived ethical misconduct can be extremely trying for psychologists involved in forensic practice activities. The following sections provide a framework for addressing perceived ethical misconduct of colleagues. The framework represents the application and adaptation of the ideas of several colleagues and of the authors (Deidan & Bush, 2002; Grote, Lewin, Sweet, & van Gorp, 2000; Martelli, Bush, & Zasler, 2003) to the current context. Exhibit 7.1 provides the framework in a checklist format for easy reference when facing possible ethical misconduct by other psychologists.

Identify the Problem

Psychologists may at times have a sense that something is "wrong" with the professional behavior of a colleague. Clearly identifying the problem or dilemma is the necessary first step to addressing it.

Consider the Relevant Ethical Issues

Psychological practices that may initially appear to be ethically questionable may instead reflect acceptable variations in practice or in the understanding of a psychological issue or condition. Before reporting allegedly unethical practice, psychologists should attempt to identify the relevant

EXHIBIT 7.1
Checklist for Reporting Ethical Violations

- Identify the problem.
- Consider the relevant ethical issues.
- Consider applicable laws and regulations.
- Consider the significance of the context and setting.
- Consider the obligations owed to the examinee/patient, referral source, and others.
- Consider the significance of the violation.
- Consider the reliability and persuasiveness of the evidence.
- Consult colleagues or ethics committees.
- Consider the possible courses of action.
- Consider the timing of any action.
- Consider the possible effects of any action or inaction.
- Consider personal beliefs, values, and feelings regarding the behavior and the colleague.
- Choose and implement a course of action, if needed.
- Assess the outcome of action or inaction and follow-up as needed.
- Document the process.

ethical issues and their specific representation in the American Psychological Association's (APA's) Ethics Code (2002) or other ethical guidelines. A lack of mention of a suspect practice does not necessarily mean that no ethical concern exists. The practice may be questionable when understood in terms of aspirational ethical principles. In such instances, open and constructive dialogue with the colleague may serve to educate one or both parties regarding a preferred manner of practice. As we have attempted to convey, there are a number of relevant sources of ethical authority that may guide forensic psychologists in their ethical, professional, legal, and moral decision making. Psychologists should avail themselves of all of these resources when attempting to clarify the ethical issues relevant to a specific situation.

Consider Applicable Laws and Regulations

State licensing laws establish regulations for the practice of psychology. State laws also mandate that particular practices be followed, such as reporting child abuse. Other state and federal laws, legal decisions, and regulations may provide further guidance regarding acceptable practice parameters.

Consider the Significance of the Context and Setting

The importance of considering context and setting in addressing perceived ethical misconduct in forensic psychology cannot be overstated. Relevant factors differ both across and within the primary practice activities and populations served. As a result, there are many parameters for ethical practice. Psychologists judging the appropriateness of colleagues' work must consider that differences in practices may reflect the different demands or allowances of the specific context. At the same time, some ethical issues transcend context and setting and must be applied universally. If unsure of the requirements of a specific setting, consult with appropriate colleagues.

Consider the Obligations Owed to the Examinee–Patient, Referral Source, and Others

Early in the process of addressing ethical misconduct, it is necessary to consider the parties to whom obligations are owed. For example, determination of who holds the privilege regarding communications may dictate the manner in which the concern is addressed. The purpose and nature of the service provided, the retaining party or referral source, and the context in which the service was provided also have implications for how ethical misconduct is addressed.

Consider the Significance of the Violation

Forensic psychologists use differing practices in establishing and maintaining professional relationships, obtaining examinee data, interpreting data, managing records, and performing other professional activities. Such differences are not necessarily problematic or indicative of failure to maintain adequate standard of care. As Blau (1998) stated, "Variations will undoubtedly occur, but they should stand the tests of being in the client's best interests and falling well within the expectancies and constraints of professional ethics, the law, and standards for the delivery of professional services" (p. 29). In addition, differences in professional practices may serve the constructive function of contributing to the advancement of the field. However, behaviors that fall well beyond the usual and customary standards of practice likely justify further examination and concern. A primary consideration is the severity of the potential misconduct.

Shuman and Greenberg (1998) examined distinctions between ethical rules in the context of admissibility decisions. However, their observation that ethical rules vary in their significance according to context pertains to the broad topic of addressing perceived ethical misconduct of colleagues. The following distinctions were offered:

> Ethical rules addressing advertising or form of practice, for example, have little bearing on the reliability of the resulting professional's information and therefore, violations of these rules should have little bearing, if any, on admissibility decisions. Ethical rules addressing integrity,

objectivity/independence, or diligence/due care, for example, have a significant impact on the reliability of the resulting professional information and therefore, violations of these rules should have a significant bearing on admissibility decisions. The ethical rules that require psychiatrists and psychologists to avoid conflicting roles ... are examples of rules that have a significant effect on the reliability of the resulting professional information, and for which unexcused violations should have a significant impact of admissibility decisions. (p. 9)

The degree of potential harmfulness of ethical misconduct will determine whether the resolution is formal or informal, and whether the misconduct is addressed prior to the completion of a legal case or following case resolution.

Consider the Reliability and Persuasiveness of the Evidence

Information and documentation observed or obtained directly by the psychologist is more reliable and persuasive than is information that is obtained secondhand. During adversarial proceedings, information obtained second hand may be intentionally or unintentionally misrepresented because of self-serving motivations of the person reporting the information. Forensic psychologists are advised to be critical of the information provided by examinees, patients, attorneys, and opposing experts. To increase the reliability and persuasiveness of the information, forensic psychologists should attempt to independently establish its accuracy (Heilbrun, Warren, & Picarello, 2003; Specialty Guidelines for Forensic Psychologists [SGFP] IV, F, Relationships; Committee on Ethical Guidelines for Forensic Psychologists, 1991).

Consult Colleagues or Ethics Committees

Consultation with colleagues or ethics committees is fundamental to addressing ethical misconduct. Such consultation may be of value at each step in the process. It is advisable to request permission from the colleagues or committees to document and cite by source their consultation (Martindale & Gould, 2004) and to ask them to maintain a record of the consultation as well.

Consider the Possible Courses of Action

When the behavior of a colleague appears to reflect ethical misconduct, the action to be taken must be carefully considered (Deidan & Bush, 2002; Grote et al., 2000; Martelli et al., 2003). As the Introduction and Applicability section of the APA Ethics Code indicates, psychologists in the process of making decisions regarding professional behavior must consider the Ethics Code, applicable laws, and psychology board regulations. They may also consider other guidelines that have been endorsed by psychological organizations, the dictates of their own conscience, and advice from colleagues.

Potential actions that psychologists may take to address perceived ethical misconduct include informal resolution that, depending on the nature of the apparent violation and any confidentiality restrictions, is generally the preferred first step (Standard 1.04, Informal Resolution of Ethical Violations). In cases of substantial harm or when informal resolution has been ineffective or would be otherwise inappropriate, further action would be required (Standard 1.05, Reporting Ethical Violations). Such actions include filing reports with institutional authorities, ethics committees that have adjudicative authority, or state licensing boards. In all cases, confidentiality restrictions should be considered. The psychologist may choose to work with the individual who holds the privilege to pursue the appropriate action.

Consider the Timing of Any Action

Having one's professional opinions aggressively challenged during adversarial proceedings may understandably result in strong emotional reactions, prompting one to interpret such challenges as unethical personal attacks. It may be natural to want to address such attacks immediately. However, the risk of addressing perceived ethical misconduct before the conclusion of a case lies in the possibility of real or perceived specious reporting designed to tarnish the credibility of the other expert (American Academy of Clinical Neuropsychology, 2003). In addition, the intensity of negative personal feelings toward a colleague and the perceived importance of the ethical issues may dissipate following conclusion of the proceedings. Thus, except for egregious ethical violations, it is often preferable to postpone ethics complaints until the conclusion of any adversarial proceedings that could benefit the complainant (American Academy of Clinical Neuropsychology, 2003). Filing ethics complaints as a litigation strategy to remove an opposing expert from a case is clearly unethical (Standard 1.07, Improper Complaints). As Nagy (2000) stated, "The ultimate purpose of filing a complaint is to protect someone from harm, not to 'get even' with another psychologist" (p. 206) or to manipulate the other psychologist in some fashion.

Consider the Possible Effects of Any Action or Inaction

The goal of addressing apparent ethical misconduct is to end or correct the misconduct. However, taking such action may have other consequences as well. Filing a complaint with an ethics committee or a state psychology board may result in counterfiling of a complaint against the psychologists who made the initial complaint. Filing a complaint may also result in litigation against the complainant for slander or defamation of character. Complaints filed during the case in which the inappropriate behavior occurred may be seen as an attempt to discredit the opposing expert, thus having the effect of discrediting the complainant and weakening the case of the party that retained the complainant. Although psychologists may have an obligation to report apparent ethical misconduct (Association of State and Provincial Psychology Boards [ASPPB], 2001, J.4.), consideration of the potential consequences of such action is prudent.

Failure to address ethical misconduct, when appropriate client authorization has been given or is not required, may result in continued harm to the recipients of psychological services, to the public, and to the profession of psychology. For those states subject to the rules of the ASPPB Code of Conduct, failure to report a violation of the statutes or rules of the Board, when there exists substantial reason to believe that such a violation has occurred, is itself a violation of the Code of Conduct. In addition, failure to address suspected ethical misconduct is counter to the General Principles of the APA Ethics Code.

Consider Personal Beliefs, Values, and Feelings Regarding the Behavior and the Colleague

Psychologists may have strong feelings about various sections of the APA Ethics Code and about other practices that are not specifically addressed by the Ethics Code. When such practices are performed in a manner that seems to be inappropriate, it may be natural to want to react forcefully. Such feelings may serve an important mobilizing function, but they may also skew one's perspective. Situations in which strong personal feelings are experienced may be those in which consultation with colleagues may be particularly beneficial.

In addition to examining personal feelings toward the ethical issues, forensic psychologists have an obligation to examine their feelings toward colleagues whose work they are reviewing or toward whom allegations of ethical misconduct may be made. The adversarial nature of forensic work may result in contentious relationships with colleagues. Reviews of one's work may be perceived as being, or may actually become, personal attacks. It may be natural for psychologists to want to respond in kind. However, forensic psychologists must strive to maintain a distinction between their feelings toward the work of colleagues and the colleagues themselves.

Choose and Implement a Course of Action, if Needed

Determine whether action is necessary. If action is deemed necessary, implement the course of action at the appropriate time. Prepare for any anticipated responses or reactions.

Assess the Outcome of Action or Inaction and Follow Up as Needed

Assess the effects of any action or inaction. If the issue was addressed, evaluate the manner in which the colleague or the relevant organization responded to the action taken. Consider and implement additional or alternative courses of action as needed to bring a satisfactory resolution to the issue.

Document the Process

Detailed documentation of each step in the process is essential to (a) explicate the rationale and procedures underlying decisions to report, or not report, perceived ethical misconduct of colleagues and (b) help clarify the psychologist's internal process so that the psychologist can use the experience to address future questions of ethical misconduct by colleagues.

CASE 6: REPORTING ETHICAL VIOLATIONS IN
FAMILY LAW MATTERS

A psychologist accepts court appointment to evaluate the mother, father, and 4-year-old daughter in a disputed custody matter following marital dissolution. The psychologist learns that the mother had been taking the child to a privately retained psychologist for "play therapy, to see if something may have happened to her," because she was exhibiting signs of distress following visits with the father. She was reportedly fussy, clingy, and demanding; was having nightmares; and was exhibiting odd behavior toward the mother and her boyfriend. Specifically, she was trying to catch glimpses of her mother's boyfriend's "privates" as he came out of the shower following afternoon swimming at their home, and she was trying to pull her mother's blouse down to expose her breast. Finally, her mother had observed her playing with her "privates" at bath time, and even saw her trying to insert a toy boat in her vagina.

The psychologist who was seeing the child in play therapy offers testimony that sexual abuse had occurred to this child, as evidenced by these symptoms and by her drawings, in play therapy, of her family in which her father was drawn with heavy, shaded lines and her mother and she were drawn more normally. She also played roughly with the anatomically detailed dolls the therapist had introduced into the play therapy to facilitate her discussions with the child of what might have happened to her. In the first six play therapy sessions, the child had insisted nothing had happened to hurt her during visitation with her father, but as she grew increasingly more comfortable with the therapist, she "opened up, and finally revealed the abuse." She said her dad had touched her "private" when drying her after her bath, when her parents first separated, and thus, when she had just turned 2 years of age. She reported he had not done that since she turned 3 years old.

On the basis of these findings, the play therapist testifies that the child should not visit the father without supervision. She had not evaluated the father or the mother, and her treatment of the child consisted of 13 play therapy sessions. She had met with the mother first individually, for an intake session, and then before and after each session, briefly in the waiting room to hear reports of the child's behavior or to report to the mother what had transpired in therapy. The father's effort to meet with her, when he learned she was treating his child, had been rebuffed; she indicates she did not believe it would be appropriate as her office was the child's "safe place" and she preferred to protect the boundaries.

The court-appointed psychologist evaluator becomes aware of this testimony after the judge rules on the matter. The judge apparently rejected the testimony of the play therapist psychologist and ordered continuation of the parents' sharing responsibility for and time with the child. She further ordered that the child not be taken to the play therapist for further sessions. The mother is to undergo some classes and individual didactic sessions to address her growing hostility toward the father, exhibited in ways evidenced by other testimony the judge heard. The court essentially made a finding that the child's best interest would be served by no further exploration of the allegation of sexual abuse.

Analysis

Identify the Problem

The court-appointed psychologist believed that the treating therapist's professional conduct was inappropriate. The primary problem was that the therapist overstepped the bounds of her treating relationship to offer testimony regarding the specific legal question. In doing so, she offered opinions and recommendations that far exceeded the information and data on which they were reportedly based. The therapist's training and experience in child therapy, particularly in the context of litigation, also came into question.

Faced with unacceptable professional conduct on the part of another psychologist, the court-appointed psychologist considered whether to file a board complaint or an ethics complaint.

Consider the Relevant Ethical Issues

The psychologist play therapist's behavior had the potential to significantly harm members of the family and their relationships (General Principle A, Beneficence and Nonmaleficence; Standard 3.04, Avoiding Harm). Offering misleading information, however unintentional, to the court had the potential to result in an inappropriate custody determination (General Principle D, Justice).

The play therapist's work was not based on established scientific and professional knowledge of child custody work (Standard 2.04, Bases for Scientific and Professional Judgments). The *Guidelines for Child Custody Evaluations in Divorce Proceedings* (APA, 1994) state in part, "Although comprehensive child custody evaluations generally require an evaluation of all parents or guardians and children, as well as observations of interactions between them, the scope of the assessment in a particular case may be limited to evaluating the parental capacity of one parent without attempting to compare the parents or to make recommendations" (III, Procedural Guidelines: Conducting a Child Custody Evaluation, § 8). The play therapist clearly failed to perform the necessary evaluations or to appropriately limit her testimony (Standard 2.01, Boundaries of Competence).

Consider Applicable Laws and Regulations

The administrative rules of practice for psychologists in the state essentially echoed the APA Ethics Code, identifying as substandard practice the offering of an opinion without benefit of adequate data.

Consider the Significance of the Context and Setting

The psychologist play therapist, working in an agency setting in which the mission of the agency was to provide assessment and treatment of abused children, was clear in testifying that her agency policy was to accept what children alleged at face value, without questioning alternative hypotheses, and then work to ensure the safety of and provide treatment for the child alleging abuse. Within that context and setting, there may have been general support for the standard of care she provided. Within the context of the courtroom, however, in which some degree of objectivity, suspended judgment, and convergence of data are sought, the care provided to the child by the play therapist psychologist may have fallen far below the standard. Questionable treatment competence, however, was not the court-appointed psychologist's primary concern. Although the court-appointed psychologist felt that "context" of the agency treatment setting might justify the play therapist's advocacy stance in the therapy room, it did not mitigate the egregiousness of the apparent violation regarding making recommendations to the court without adequate data.

Consider the Obligations Owed to the Examinee–Patient, Referral Source, and Others

The court had already essentially dismissed the testimony and recommendations of the treating therapist. As a result, the child and the family were presumably not permanently harmed by the actions of the therapist, in offering unsubstantiated opinion in court. Nevertheless, the potential for the therapist to perform similarly in another case remained. Therefore, the court-appointed psychologist considered her obligations to the legal system and the public. She had an obligation to protect the legal system and society from the potential harm that could be caused by a psychologist practicing beyond her area of expertise and competence. The court-appointed psychologist also had an obligation to the profession of psychology to take action when one of its members tarnished the credibility of the profession in the courtroom, with the family, and beyond.

Consider the Significance of the Violation

The court-appointed psychologist considered the treating therapist's ethical violations to be significant. In the transparent setting of the courtroom, and in an adversarial proceeding, there was a good opportunity for the allegedly unethical behavior to yield its just due—lessening the credibility of the wrongdoer and invoking, in the end, an outcome unfavorable to the play therapist psychologist's apparent intention. That the litigants may have suffered terribly, in the process, and the profession of psychology was harmed by the egregious behavior of the play therapist was almost certain. Clearly, further action was warranted to discharge the court-appointed psychologist's ethical responsibility to uphold the values of nonmaleficence and justice. The case did not, at this point, involve a civil action against the alleged offender for failure to meet the standard of care (and if it had, then the court-appointed psychologist would have had no responsibility to report, in that the standard of practice issue was to be decided by the court, and the alleged victim could enjoy some redress. Further, the play therapist, having been sued for practicing below the standard of care, would then have been obligated to report the court action to the state board).

Consider the Reliability and Persuasiveness of the Evidence

The court-appointed psychologist believed that she had strong evidence of the professional misconduct. In addition to the potentially less reliable verbal reports of those involved in the case, she received a copy of, and carefully reviewed, the court transcript of the play therapist's testimony.

Consult Colleagues or Ethics Committees

Before consulting with colleagues or filing a report with any authority, the psychologist first addressed the issue of confidentiality. The case had been heard in court, and the testimony of the play therapist psychologist was a matter of public record, so no confidentiality concerns existed.

Upon consultation with colleagues, the psychologist learned that (a) the play therapist had been previously sanctioned by the state board for offering an opinion about the diagnosis of a party without benefit of evaluation or review of prior treatment records and (b) the alleged offender had attended a continuing education workshop conducted by one of the colleagues consulted in this matter within the past year and had received clear instruction about the inappropriateness of making custody or access recommendations without examining one of the parties (handouts for the workshop having included Otto, Buffington-Vollum, & Edens, 2002; the APA Ethics Code; the APA *Guidelines for Child Custody Evaluations in Divorce Proceedings*; and the SGFP). Colleagues opined that it was the duty of the court-appointed psychologist to report the play therapist's actions to the board and to the APA Ethics Committee.

Consider the Possible Courses of Action

Consultation of appropriate authoritative sources left the forensic psychologist convinced of the following:

1. It was necessary to take some action. Although the state board rules did not require that a complaint be filed, and consultation with their counsel suggested that without the injured party filing a complaint it was likely that the matter would not be investigated, the APA Ethics Code did support the importance of taking appropriate action, including referral to state or national committees on professional ethics, to state licensing boards, or to the appropriate institutional authorities.
2. Owing to the somewhat less-than-extreme nature of the apparent wrongdoing, it might be preferable to approach the play therapist directly with the concern before taking the matter further (more outrageous action might include engaging in a felonious criminal action, such as sexual exploitation of a patient, sexual abuse of a child, extorting money from a patient, filing insurance claims for parties never seen, and so on; Standard 1.04, Informal Resolution of Ethical Violations).

Consider the Timing of Any Action

Aware that allegations of professional misconduct made during the course of litigation may raise questions about the reporting psychologist's motivations, the court-appointed psychologist was sensitive to the importance of timing of any action. The timing, following the culmination of the hearing, was appropriate in that the consultation with the alleged offender would likely not be construed as witness tampering or other attempted manipulation of the case outcome.

Consider the Possible Effects of Any Action or Inaction

Ideally, the treating psychologist would be open to education from the court-appointed psychologist about the need to appropriately limit testimony. However, because the treating psychologist had received such information before and had in fact been formally sanctioned, the court-appointed psychologist was concerned that informal resolution would not have the intended effect of protecting those who could be harmed from future misconduct. However, the court-appointed psychologist was confident that failure to act could only result in further misconduct. The filing of a formal complaint may have greater potential to achieve the desire goal of protecting the public; however, it may also interfere with clients of the agency receiving much-needed clinical services. Such a filing may also result in a charge of libel by the treating psychologist.

Consider Personal Beliefs, Values, and Feelings Regarding the Behavior and the Colleague

The court-appointed psychologist had strong personal convictions that zealous advocacy of a stance could interfere with professional objectivity. Perceiving the play therapist to potentially suffer from clouded judgment in the matter at hand, the court-appointed psychologist had to weigh whether impatience with that posture was motivating a state board or ethics complaint. Holding a personal belief that children are often harmed by such intervention, there was a tendency toward outrage that a terrible wrong may have been perpetrated to the child and the parent if the accusation of sexual abuse was unfounded. It would have been easy to displace some aggressive energy to the process of filing a complaint, and the psychologist gave consideration to this issue.

Choose and Implement a Course of Action, if Needed

It was clear that the alleged offender had already been put on notice that the act of making unsubstantiated custody recommendations was below the standard of care for psychologists and, nevertheless, had engaged in this action. The court-appointed psychologist anticipated no benefit from attempting to resolve the problem by bringing it to the play therapist's attention. She recognized that although the behavior did not represent a direct threat to the physical safety of another, it might well constitute a serious challenge to the well-being of others in the long run. Because of these factors and the risk of recurrence, the psychologist saw an absolute obligation to report the offense to the state licensing board.

There was no reason for the psychologist to attempt to invoke a companion complaint from the allegedly injured party, although the state board staff counsel indicated, when the psychologist called to inquire about making a report, that it would be easier to investigate if that were done. The potential for a charge of libel did not warrant its possible benefit, given that there was a court transcript available to document the alleged wrong, and the psychologist was able to obtain it and provide it to the state board to supplement the complaint. A complaint to the APA Ethics Committee was also warranted. Standard 1.05, Reporting Ethical Violations, of the APA Ethics Code states,

> If an apparent ethical violation has substantially harmed or is likely to substantially harm a person or organization and is not appropriate for informal resolution under Standard 1.04, Informal Resolution of Ethical Violations, or is not resolved properly in that fashion, psychologists take further action appropriate to the situation. Such action might include referral to state or national committees on professional ethics, to state licensing boards, or to the appropriate institutional authorities. This standard does not apply when an intervention would violate confidentiality rights or when psychologists have been retained to review the work of another psychologist whose professional conduct is in question.

However, a review of the APA membership directory revealed that the play therapist was not an APA member. Therefore, APA could not impose sanctions, if indicated, on the alleged offender.

Assess the Outcome of Action or Inaction and Follow Up as Needed

Having filed complaints with the state licensing board and the APA Ethics Committee, the court-appointed psychologist found that there was little else that could be done to ensure that the alleged offender would adhere to the ethical standards and guidelines admonishing the withholding of an unsubstantiated opinion. The outcome of the complaint process was that the play therapist psychologist was again sanctioned by the state board, but she shortly moved out of the area, so the court-appointed psychologist did not have further interaction with her. The process of researching options, including especially the collegial consultations, proved time consuming but educative, and the psychologist recognized that further action might generate liability without an increasing probability of successful resolution. There was the further possibility that through the adversarial process of the family courts, the alleged offender's actions would continue to elicit the natural consequence of reduced credibility, and although vulnerable individuals might nevertheless be deprived of just services, the overarching value of justice would likely prevail.

Document the Process

The court-appointed psychologist maintained detailed documentation of all consultation-related matters involving this case, including the steps taken once the potential professional and ethical misconduct was detected. The thorough documentation served her particularly well when she filed the complaints.

AFTERWORD

Competent, ethical psychologists provide a valuable service to the justice system; however, the practice of forensic psychology is susceptible to ethical misconduct on many fronts, from unintentional missteps to strong enticements to sacrifice moral principles. Maintaining professional competence and ethical behavior requires a lifelong commitment to high moral standards and continuing education. We believe that in the abstract, nearly all psychologists would embrace a commitment to the highest standards of ethical practice. However, embracing a commitment to ethical practice in the abstract, such as while one is having coffee and reading the newspaper in the morning (if the demanding life of a psychologist still allows time for such things), is quite different from embracing such a commitment when faced with a persuasive attorney or considerable financial incentive.

Forensic psychologists must reaffirm their commitment to the highest standards of ethical practice not just when practice is going smoothly but particularly when faced with enticement to ethical misconduct. Such enticements may take many forms, such as receiving a referral for which professional competence may be lacking or the promise of remuneration for offering opinions that lack proper support. For example, forensic psychologists may, at some point, experience something similar to the following:

> An attorney calls and says,
> "I received your report. It was great. Thanks very much. I'm putting your check in the mail right now, and I want to talk to you about a couple of new cases, but first, I have a question about that last sentence of your report. Would you mind changing the statement ' . . . and seems to be disabled due to the emotional distress that emerged or worsened following the accident' to ' . . . is permanently disabled as a result of the accident'?"

It is precisely when psychologists consider engaging in professional conduct that they suspect or know to be ethically inappropriate, or their colleagues may consider ethically questionable, that they must reaffirm their commitment to high ethical standards of practice.

Although the financial temptations associated with forensic practice may at times represent the most obvious and most emphasized threats to ethical practice, psychologists in forensic practice face ethical challenges on many fronts. The challenges associated with becoming and remaining knowledgeable about ethical standards and guidelines, overcoming personal biases, and recognizing the potential for harm, are equally important.

A proactive approach to ethical practice may help to reduce the occurrence of, or problems that arise from, ethical dilemmas. In addition to continuing education, forensic psychologists are advised to pursue informal peer consultation that focuses specifically on professional ethics. For example, psychologists may find it beneficial to periodically send a copy of a report to a respected colleague, asking that the report be reviewed for the existence of ethically questionable statements or practices. Honest, objective feedback about one's practices can help to refine behaviors so that high ethical standards of practice are maintained. Although agreement among forensic psychologists, including those who present and write about ethics, regarding what constitutes ethical practice in all situations is not unanimous, obtaining the perspectives of colleagues can be of considerable value in avoiding ethical misconduct.

Forensic psychologists bear a considerable responsibility to individuals, institutions, and society. Once a commitment to maintaining the highest ethical standards has been affirmed, written and collegial resources can help psychologists negotiate the unique details of a given ethical challenge. The practice of forensic psychology can be both challenging and rewarding; perhaps the greatest challenge is in keeping one's values in perspective.

APPENDIX:
Ethical Principles of Psychologists and Code of Conduct

CONTENTS

Introduction and Applicability

Preamble

General Principles

ETHICAL STANDARDS

From "Ethical Principles of Psychologists and Code of Conduct," by the American Psychological Association, 2002, *American Psychologist, 57*, pp. 1597–1611. Copyright 2002 by the American Psychological Association. Also available from the PsychNET Web site: http://www.apa.org/ethics/code2002.html

Introduction and Applicability

The American Psychological Association's (APA's) Ethical Principles of Psychologists and Code of Conduct (hereinafter referred to as the Ethics Code) consists of an Introduction, a Preamble, five General Principles (A–E), and specific Ethical Standards. The Introduction discusses the intent, organization, procedural considerations, and scope of application of the Ethics Code. The Preamble and General Principles are aspirational goals to guide psychologists toward the highest ideals of psychology. Although the Preamble and General Principles are not themselves enforceable rules, they should be considered by psychologists in arriving at an ethical course of action. The Ethical Standards set forth enforceable rules for conduct as psychologists. Most of the Ethical Standards are written broadly, in order to apply to psychologists in varied roles, although the application of an Ethical Standard

---

This version of the APA Ethics Code was adopted by the American Psychological Association's Council of Representatives during its meeting, August 21, 2002, and is effective beginning June 1, 2003. Inquiries concerning the substance or interpretation of the APA Ethics Code should be addressed to the Director, Office of Ethics, American Psychological Association, 750 First Street, NE, Washington, DC 20002-4242. The Ethics Code and information regarding the Code can be found on the APA Web site, http://www.apa.org/ethics. The standards in this Ethics Code will be used to adjudicate complaints brought concerning alleged conduct occurring on or after the effective date. Complaints regarding conduct occurring prior to the effective date will be adjudicated on the basis of the version of the Ethics Code that was in effect at the time the conduct occurred.

may vary depending on the context. The Ethical Standards are not exhaustive. The fact that a given conduct is not specifically addressed by an Ethical Standard does not mean that it is necessarily either ethical or unethical.

This Ethics Code applies only to psychologists' activities that are part of their scientific, educational, or professional roles as psychologists. Areas covered include but are not limited to the clinical, counseling, and school practice of psychology; research; teaching; supervision of trainees; public service; policy development; social intervention; development of assessment instruments; conducting assessments; educational counseling; organizational consulting; forensic activities; program design and evaluation; and administration. This Ethics Code applies to these activities across a variety of contexts, such as in person, postal, telephone, Internet, and other electronic transmissions. These activities shall be distinguished from the purely private conduct of psychologists, which is not within the purview of the Ethics Code.

Membership in the APA commits members and student affiliates to comply with the standards of the APA Ethics Code and to the rules and procedures used to enforce them. Lack of awareness or misunderstanding of an Ethical Standard is not itself a defense to a charge of unethical conduct.

The procedures for filing, investigating, and resolving complaints of unethical conduct are described in the current Rules and Procedures of the APA Ethics Committee. APA may impose sanctions on its members for violations of the standards of the Ethics Code, including termination of APA membership, and may notify other bodies and individuals of its actions. Actions that violate the standards of the Ethics Code may also lead to the imposition of sanctions on psychologists or students whether or not they are APA members by bodies other than APA, including state psychological associations, other professional groups, psychology boards, other state or federal agencies, and payors for health services. In addition, APA may take action against a member after his or her conviction of a felony, expulsion or suspension from an affiliated state psychological association, or suspension or loss of licensure. When the sanction to be imposed by APA is less than expulsion, the 2001 Rules and Procedures do not guarantee an opportunity for an in-person hearing, but generally provide that complaints will be resolved only on the basis of a submitted record.

The Ethics Code is intended to provide guidance for psychologists and standards of professional conduct that can be applied by the APA and by other bodies that choose to adopt them. The Ethics Code is not intended to be a basis of civil liability. Whether a psychologist has violated the Ethics Code standards does not by itself determine whether the psychologist is legally liable in a court action, whether a contract is enforceable, or whether other legal consequences occur.

The modifiers used in some of the standards of this Ethics Code (e.g., *reasonably*, *appropriate*, *potentially*) are included in the standards when they would (1) allow professional judgment on the part of psychologists, (2) eliminate injustice or inequality that would occur without the modifier, (3) ensure applicability across the broad range of activities conducted by psychologists, or (4) guard against a set of rigid rules that might be quickly outdated. As used in this Ethics Code, the term *reasonable* means the prevailing professional judgment of psychologists engaged in similar activities in similar circumstances, given the knowledge the psychologist had or should have had at the time.

In the process of making decisions regarding their professional behavior, psychologists must consider this Ethics Code in addition to applicable laws and psychology board regulations. In applying the Ethics Code to their professional work, psychologists may consider other materials and guidelines that have been adopted or endorsed by scientific and professional psychological organizations and the dictates of their own conscience, as well as consult with others within the field. If this Ethics Code establishes a higher standard of conduct than is required by law, psychologists must meet the higher ethical standard. If psychologists' ethical responsibilities conflict with law, regulations, or other governing legal authority, psychologists make known their commitment to this Ethics Code and take steps to resolve the conflict in a responsible manner. If the conflict is unresolvable via such means, psychologists may adhere to the requirements of the law, regulations, or other governing authority in keeping with basic principles of human rights.

Preamble

Psychologists are committed to increasing scientific and professional knowledge of behavior and people's understanding of themselves and others and to the use of such knowledge to improve the condition of individuals, organizations, and society. Psychologists respect and protect civil and human rights and the central importance of freedom of inquiry and expression in research, teaching, and publication. They strive to help the public in developing informed judgments and choices concerning human behavior. In doing so, they perform many roles, such as researcher, educator, diagnostician, therapist, supervisor, consultant, administrator, social interventionist, and expert witness. This Ethics Code provides a common set of principles and standards upon which psychologists build their professional and scientific work.

This Ethics Code is intended to provide specific standards to cover most situations encountered by psychologists. It has as its goals the welfare and protection of the individuals and groups with whom psychologists work and the education of members, students, and the public regarding ethical standards of the discipline.

The development of a dynamic set of ethical standards for psychologists' work-related conduct requires a personal commitment and lifelong effort to act ethically; to encourage ethical behavior by students, supervisees, employees, and colleagues; and to consult with others concerning ethical problems.

General Principles

This section consists of General Principles. General Principles, as opposed to Ethical Standards, are aspirational in nature. Their intent is to guide and inspire psychologists toward the very highest ethical ideals of the profession. General Principles, in contrast to Ethical Standards, do not represent obligations and should not form the basis for imposing sanctions. Relying upon General Principles for either of these reasons distorts both their meaning and purpose.

Principle A: Beneficence and Nonmaleficence. Psychologists strive to benefit those with whom they work and take care to do no harm. In their professional actions, psychologists seek to safeguard the welfare and rights of those with whom they interact professionally and other affected persons, and the welfare of animal subjects of research. When conflicts occur among psychologists' obligations or concerns, they attempt to resolve these conflicts in a responsible fashion that avoids or minimizes harm. Because psychologists' scientific and professional judgments and actions may affect the lives of others, they are alert to and guard against personal, financial, social, organizational, or political factors that might lead to misuse of their influence. Psychologists strive to be aware of the possible effect of their own physical and mental health on their ability to help those with whom they work.

Principle B: Fidelity and Responsibility. Psychologists establish relationships of trust with those with whom they work. They are aware of their professional and scientific responsibilities to society and to the specific communities in which they work. Psychologists uphold professional standards of conduct, clarify their professional roles and obligations, accept appropriate responsibility for their behavior, and seek to manage conflicts of interest that could lead to exploitation or harm. Psychologists consult with, refer to, or cooperate with other professionals and institutions to the extent needed to serve the best interests of those with whom they work. They are concerned about the ethical compliance of their colleagues' scientific and professional conduct. Psychologists strive to contribute a portion of their professional time for little or no compensation or personal advantage.

Principle C: Integrity. Psychologists seek to promote accuracy, honesty, and truthfulness in the science, teaching, and practice of psychology. In these activities psychologists do not steal, cheat, or engage in fraud, subterfuge, or intentional misrepresentation of fact. Psychologists strive to keep their promises and to avoid unwise or unclear commitments. In situations in which deception may be ethically justifiable to maximize benefits and minimize harm, psychologists have a serious obligation to consider the need for, the possible consequences of, and their responsibility to correct any resulting mistrust or other harmful effects that arise from the use of such techniques.

Principle D: Justice. Psychologists recognize that fairness and justice entitle all persons to access to and benefit from the contributions of psychology and to equal quality in the processes, procedures, and services being conducted by psychologists. Psychologists exercise reasonable judgment and take precautions to ensure that their potential biases, the boundaries of their competence, and the limitations of their expertise do not lead to or condone unjust practices.

Principle E: Respect for People's Rights and Dignity. Psychologists respect the dignity and worth of all people, and the rights of individuals to privacy, confidentiality, and self-determination. Psychologists are aware that special safeguards may be necessary to protect the rights and welfare of persons or communities whose vulnerabilities impair autonomous decision making. Psychologists are aware of and respect cultural, individual, and role differences, including those based on age, gender, gender identity, race, ethnicity, culture, national origin, religion, sexual orientation, disability, language, and socioeconomic status and consider these factors when working with members of such groups. Psychologists try to eliminate the effect on their work of biases based on those factors, and they do not knowingly participate in or condone activities of others based upon such prejudices.

Ethical Standards

1. Resolving Ethical Issues

1.01 Misuse of Psychologists' Work. If psychologists learn of misuse or misrepresentation of their work, they take reasonable steps to correct or minimize the misuse or misrepresentation.

1.02 Conflicts Between Ethics and Law, Regulations, or Other Governing Legal Authority. If psychologists' ethical responsibilities conflict with law, regulations, or other governing legal authority, psychologists make known their commitment to the Ethics Code and take steps to resolve the conflict. If the conflict is unresolvable via such means, psychologists may adhere to the requirements of the law, regulations, or other governing legal authority.

1.03 Conflicts Between Ethics and Organizational Demands. If the demands of an organization with which psychologists are affiliated or for whom they are working conflict with this Ethics Code, psychologists clarify the nature of the conflict, make known their commitment to the Ethics Code, and to the extent feasible, resolve the conflict in a way that permits adherence to the Ethics Code.

1.04 Informal Resolution of Ethical Violations. When psychologists believe that there may have been an ethical violation by another psychologist, they attempt to resolve the issue by bringing it to the attention of that individual, if an informal resolution appears appropriate and the intervention does not violate any confidentiality rights that may be involved. (See also Standards 1.02, Conflicts Between Ethics and Law, Regulations, or Other Governing Legal Authority, and 1.03, Conflicts Between Ethics and Organizational Demands.)

1.05 Reporting Ethical Violations. If an apparent ethical violation has substantially harmed or is likely to substantially harm a person or organization and is not appropriate for informal resolution under Standard 1.04, Informal Resolution of Ethical Violations, or is not resolved properly in that fashion, psychologists take further action appropriate to the situation. Such action might include referral to state or national committees on professional ethics, to state licensing boards, or to the appropriate institutional authorities. This standard does not apply when an intervention would violate confidentiality rights or when psychologists have been retained to review the work of another psychologist whose professional conduct is in question. (See also Standard 1.02, Conflicts Between Ethics and Law, Regulations, or Other Governing Legal Authority.)

1.06 Cooperating With Ethics Committees. Psychologists cooperate in ethics investigations, proceedings, and resulting requirements of the APA or any affiliated state psychological association to which they belong. In doing so, they address any confidentiality issues. Failure to cooperate is itself an ethics violation. However, making a request for deferment of adjudication of an ethics complaint pending the outcome of litigation does not alone constitute noncooperation.

1.07 Improper Complaints. Psychologists do not file or encourage the filing of ethics complaints that are made with reckless disregard for or willful ignorance of facts that would disprove the allegation.

1.08 Unfair Discrimination Against Complainants and Respondents. Psychologists do not deny persons employment, advancement, admissions to academic or other programs, tenure, or promotion, based solely upon their having made or their being the subject of an ethics complaint. This does not preclude taking action based upon the outcome of such proceedings or considering other appropriate information.

2. Competence

2.01 Boundaries of Competence. (a) Psychologists provide services, teach, and conduct research with populations and in areas only within the boundaries of their competence, based on their education, training, supervised experience, consultation, study, or professional experience.

(b) Where scientific or professional knowledge in the discipline of psychology establishes that an understanding of factors associated with age, gender, gender identity, race, ethnicity, culture, national origin, religion, sexual orientation, disability, language, or socioeconomic status is essential for effective implementation of their services or research, psychologists have or obtain the training, experience, consultation, or supervision necessary to ensure the competence of their services, or they make appropriate referrals, except as provided in Standard 2.02, Providing Services in Emergencies.

(c) Psychologists planning to provide services, teach, or conduct research involving populations, areas, techniques, or technologies new to them undertake relevant education, training, supervised experience, consultation, or study.

(d) When psychologists are asked to provide services to individuals for whom appropriate mental health services are not available and for which psychologists have not obtained the competence necessary, psychologists with closely related prior training or experience may provide such services in order to ensure that services are not denied if they make a reasonable effort to obtain the competence required by using relevant research, training, consultation, or study.

(e) In those emerging areas in which generally recognized standards for preparatory training do not yet exist, psychologists nevertheless take reasonable steps to ensure the competence of their work and to protect clients/patients, students, supervisees, research participants, organizational clients, and others from harm.

(f) When assuming forensic roles, psychologists are or become reasonably familiar with the judicial or administrative rules governing their roles.

2.02 Providing Services in Emergencies. In emergencies, when psychologists provide services to individuals for whom other mental health services are not available and for which psychologists have not obtained the necessary training, psychologists may provide such services in order to ensure that services are not denied. The services are discontinued as soon as the emergency has ended or appropriate services are available.

2.03 Maintaining Competence. Psychologists undertake ongoing efforts to develop and maintain their competence.

2.04 Bases for Scientific and Professional Judgments. Psychologists' work is based upon established scientific and professional knowledge of the discipline. (See also Standards 2.01e, Boundaries of Competence, and 10.01b, Informed Consent to Therapy.)

2.05 Delegation of Work to Others. Psychologists who delegate work to employees, supervisees, or research or teaching assistants or who use the services of others, such as interpreters, take reasonable steps to (1) avoid delegating such work to persons who have a multiple relationship with those being served that would likely lead to exploitation or loss of objectivity; (2) authorize only those responsibilities that such persons can be expected to perform competently on the basis of their education, training, or experience, either independently or with the level of supervision being provided; and (3) see that such persons perform these services competently. (See also Standards 2.02, Providing Services in Emergencies; 3.05, Multiple Relationships; 4.01, Maintaining Confidentiality; 9.01, Bases for Assessments; 9.02, Use of Assessments; 9.03, Informed Consent in Assessments; and 9.07, Assessment by Unqualified Persons.)

2.06 Personal Problems and Conflicts. (a) Psychologists refrain from initiating an activity when they know or should know that there is a substantial likelihood that their personal problems will prevent them from performing their work-related activities in a competent manner.

(b) When psychologists become aware of personal problems that may interfere with their performing work-related duties adequately, they take appropriate measures, such as obtaining professional consultation or assistance, and determine whether they should limit, suspend, or terminate their work-related duties. (See also Standard 10.10, Terminating Therapy.)

3. Human Relations

3.01 Unfair Discrimination. In their work-related activities, psychologists do not engage in unfair discrimination based on age, gender, gender identity, race, ethnicity, culture, national origin, religion, sexual orientation, disability, socioeconomic status, or any basis proscribed by law.

3.02 Sexual Harassment. Psychologists do not engage in sexual harassment. Sexual harassment is sexual solicitation, physical advances, or verbal or nonverbal conduct that is sexual in nature, that occurs in connection with the psychologist's activities or roles as a psychologist, and that either (1) is unwelcome, is offensive, or creates a hostile workplace or educational environment, and the psychologist knows or is told this or (2) is sufficiently severe or intense to be abusive to a reasonable person in the context. Sexual harassment can consist of a single intense or severe act or of multiple persistent or pervasive acts. (See also Standard 1.08, Unfair Discrimination Against Complainants and Respondents.)

3.03 Other Harassment. Psychologists do not knowingly engage in behavior that is harassing or demeaning to persons with whom they interact in their work based on factors such as those persons' age, gender, gender identity, race, ethnicity, culture, national origin, religion, sexual orientation, disability, language, or socioeconomic status.

3.04 Avoiding Harm. Psychologists take reasonable steps to avoid harming their clients/patients, students, supervisees, research participants, organizational clients, and others with whom they work, and to minimize harm where it is foreseeable and unavoidable.

3.05 *Multiple Relationships.* (a) A multiple relationship occurs when a psychologist is in a professional role with a person and (1) at the same time is in another role with the same person, (2) at the same time is in a relationship with a person closely associated with or related to the person with whom the psychologist has the professional relationship, or (3) promises to enter into another relationship in the future with the person or a person closely associated with or related to the person.

A psychologist refrains from entering into a multiple relationship if the multiple relationship could reasonably be expected to impair the psychologist's objectivity, competence, or effectiveness in performing his or her functions as a psychologist, or otherwise risks exploitation or harm to the person with whom the professional relationship exists.

Multiple relationships that would not reasonably be expected to cause impairment or risk exploitation or harm are not unethical.

(b) If a psychologist finds that, due to unforeseen factors, a potentially harmful multiple relationship has arisen, the psychologist takes reasonable steps to resolve it with due regard for the best interests of the affected person and maximal compliance with the Ethics Code.

(c) When psychologists are required by law, institutional policy, or extraordinary circumstances to serve in more than one role in judicial or administrative proceedings, at the outset they clarify role expectations and the extent of confidentiality and thereafter as changes occur. (See also Standards 3.04, Avoiding Harm, and 3.07, Third-Party Requests for Services.)

3.06 *Conflict of Interest.* Psychologists refrain from taking on a professional role when personal, scientific, professional, legal, financial, or other interests or relationships could reasonably be expected to (1) impair their objectivity, competence, or effectiveness in performing their functions as psychologists or (2) expose the person or organization with whom the professional relationship exists to harm or exploitation.

3.07 *Third-Party Requests for Services.* When psychologists agree to provide services to a person or entity at the request of a third party, psychologists attempt to clarify at the outset of the service the nature of the relationship with all individuals or organizations involved. This clarification includes the role of the psychologist (e.g., therapist, consultant, diagnostician, or expert witness), an identification of who is the client, the probable uses of the services provided or the information obtained, and the fact that there may be limits to confidentiality. (See also Standards 3.05, Multiple Relationships, and 4.02, Discussing the Limits of Confidentiality.)

3.08 *Exploitative Relationships.* Psychologists do not exploit persons over whom they have supervisory, evaluative, or other authority such as clients/patients, students, supervisees, research participants, and employees. (See also Standards 3.05, Multiple Relationships; 6.04, Fees and Financial Arrangements; 6.05, Barter with Clients/Patients; 7.07, Sexual Relationships with Students and Supervisees; 10.05, Sexual Intimacies With Current Therapy Clients/Patients; 10.06, Sexual Intimacies With Relatives or Significant Others of Current Therapy Clients/Patients; 10.07, Therapy With Former Sexual Partners; and 10.08, Sexual Intimacies With Former Therapy Clients/Patients.)

3.09 Cooperation With Other Professionals. When indicated and professionally appropriate, psychologists cooperate with other professionals in order to serve their clients/patients effectively and appropriately. (See also Standard 4.05, Disclosures.)

3.10 Informed Consent. (a) When psychologists conduct research or provide assessment, therapy, counseling, or consulting services in person or via electronic transmission or other forms of communication, they obtain the informed consent of the individual or individuals using language that is reasonably understandable to that person or persons except when conducting such activities without consent is mandated by law or governmental regulation or as otherwise provided in this Ethics Code. (See also Standards 8.02, Informed Consent to Research; 9.03, Informed Consent in Assessments; and 10.01, Informed Consent to Therapy.)

(b) For persons who are legally incapable of giving informed consent, psychologists nevertheless (1) provide an appropriate explanation, (2) seek the individual's assent, (3) consider such persons' preferences and best interests, and (4) obtain appropriate permission from a legally authorized person, if such substitute consent is permitted or required by law. When consent by a legally authorized person is not permitted or required by law, psychologists take reasonable steps to protect the individual's rights and welfare.

(c) When psychological services are court ordered or otherwise mandated, psychologists inform the individual of the nature of the anticipated services, including whether the services are court ordered or mandated and any limits of confidentiality, before proceeding.

(d) Psychologists appropriately document written or oral consent, permission, and assent. (See also Standards 8.02, Informed Consent to Research; 9.03, Informed Consent in Assessments; and 10.01, Informed Consent to Therapy.)

3.11 Psychological Services Delivered to or Through Organizations. (a) Psychologists delivering services to or through organizations provide information beforehand to clients and when appropriate those directly affected by the services about (1) the nature and objectives of the services, (2) the intended recipients, (3) which of the individuals are clients, (4) the relationship the psychologist will have with each person and the organization, (5) the probable uses of services provided and information obtained, (6) who will have access to the information, and (7) limits of confidentiality. As soon as feasible, they provide information about the results and conclusions of such services to appropriate persons.

(b) If psychologists will be precluded by law or by organizational roles from providing such information to particular individuals or groups, they so inform those individuals or groups at the outset of the service.

3.12 Interruption of Psychological Services. Unless otherwise covered by contract, psychologists make reasonable efforts to plan for facilitating services in the event that psychological services are interrupted by factors such as the psychologist's illness, death, unavailability, relocation, or retirement or by the client's/patient's relocation or financial limitations. (See also Standard 6.02c, Maintenance, Dissemination, and Disposal of Confidential Records of Professional and Scientific Work.)

4. Privacy and Confidentiality

4.01 Maintaining Confidentiality. Psychologists have a primary obligation and take reasonable precautions to protect confidential information obtained through or stored in any medium, recognizing that the extent and limits of confidentiality may be regulated by law or established by institutional rules or professional or scientific relationship. (See also Standard 2.05, Delegation of Work to Others.)

4.02 Discussing the Limits of Confidentiality. (a) Psychologists discuss with persons (including, to the extent feasible, persons who are legally incapable of giving informed consent and their legal representatives) and organizations with whom they establish a scientific or professional relationship (1) the relevant limits of confidentiality and (2) the foreseeable uses of the information generated through their psychological activities. (See also Standard 3.10, Informed Consent.)

(b) Unless it is not feasible or is contraindicated, the discussion of confidentiality occurs at the outset of the relationship and thereafter as new circumstances may warrant.

(c) Psychologists who offer services, products, or information via electronic transmission inform clients/patients of the risks to privacy and limits of confidentiality.

4.03 Recording. Before recording the voices or images of individuals to whom they provide services, psychologists obtain permission from all such persons or their legal representatives. (See also Standards 8.03, Informed Consent for Recording Voices and Images in Research; 8.05, Dispensing With Informed Consent for Research; and 8.07, Deception in Research.)

4.04 *Minimizing Intrusions on Privacy.* (a) Psychologists include in written and oral reports and consultations, only information germane to the purpose for which the communication is made.

(b) Psychologists discuss confidential information obtained in their work only for appropriate scientific or professional purposes and only with persons clearly concerned with such matters.

4.05 *Disclosures.* (a) Psychologists may disclose confidential information with the appropriate consent of the organizational client, the individual client/patient, or another legally authorized person on behalf of the client/ patient unless prohibited by law.

(b) Psychologists disclose confidential information without the consent of the individual only as mandated by law, or where permitted by law for a valid purpose such as to (1) provide needed professional services; (2) obtain appropriate professional consultations; (3) protect the client/patient, psychologist, or others from harm; or (4) obtain payment for services from a client/patient, in which instance disclosure is limited to the minimum that is necessary to achieve the purpose. (See also Standard 6.04e, Fees and Financial Arrangements.)

4.06 *Consultations.* When consulting with colleagues, (1) psychologists do not disclose confidential information that reasonably could lead to the identification of a client/patient, research participant, or other person or organization with whom they have a confidential relationship unless they have obtained the prior consent of the person or organization or the disclosure cannot be avoided, and (2) they disclose information only to the extent necessary to achieve the purposes of the consultation. (See also Standard 4.01, Maintaining Confidentiality.)

4.07 *Use of Confidential Information for Didactic or Other Purposes.* Psychologists do not disclose in their writings, lectures, or other public media, confidential, personally identifiable information concerning their clients/ patients, students, research participants, organizational clients, or other recipients of their services that they obtained during the course of their work, unless (1) they take reasonable steps to disguise the person or organization, (2) the person or organization has consented in writing, or (3) there is legal authorization for doing so.

5. *Advertising and Other Public Statements*

5.01 *Avoidance of False or Deceptive Statements.* (a) Public statements include but are not limited to paid or unpaid advertising, product endorsements, grant applications, licensing applications, other credentialing applications, brochures, printed matter, directory listings, personal resumes or curricula vitae, or comments for use in media such as print or electronic transmission, statements in legal proceedings, lectures and public oral presentations, and published materials. Psychologists do not knowingly make public statements that are false, deceptive, or fraudulent concerning their research, practice, or other work activities or those of persons or organizations with which they are affiliated.

(b) Psychologists do not make false, deceptive, or fraudulent statements concerning (1) their training, experience, or competence; (2) their academic degrees; (3) their credentials; (4) their institutional or association affiliations; (5) their services; (6) the scientific or clinical basis for, or results or degree of success of, their services; (7) their fees; or (8) their publications or research findings.

(c) Psychologists claim degrees as credentials for their health services only if those degrees (1) were earned from a regionally accredited educational institution or (2) were the basis for psychology licensure by the state in which they practice.

5.02 Statements by Others. (a) Psychologists who engage others to create or place public statements that promote their professional practice, products, or activities retain professional responsibility for such statements.

(b) Psychologists do not compensate employees of press, radio, television, or other communication media in return for publicity in a news item. (See also Standard 1.01, Misuse of Psychologists' Work.)

(c) A paid advertisement relating to psychologists' activities must be identified or clearly recognizable as such.

5.03 Descriptions of Workshops and Non-Degree-Granting Educational Programs. To the degree to which they exercise control, psychologists responsible for announcements, catalogs, brochures, or advertisements describing workshops, seminars, or other non-degree-granting educational programs ensure that they accurately describe the audience for which the program is intended, the educational objectives, the presenters, and the fees involved.

5.04 Media Presentations. When psychologists provide public advice or comment via print, Internet, or other electronic transmission, they take precautions to ensure that statements (1) are based on their professional knowledge, training, or experience in accord with appropriate psychological literature and practice; (2) are otherwise consistent with this Ethics Code; and (3) do not indicate that a professional relationship has been established with the recipient. (See also Standard 2.04, Bases for Scientific and Professional Judgments.)

5.05 Testimonials. Psychologists do not solicit testimonials from current therapy clients/patients or other persons who because of their particular circumstances are vulnerable to undue influence.

5.06 In-Person Solicitation. Psychologists do not engage, directly or through agents, in uninvited in-person solicitation of business from actual or potential therapy clients/patients or other persons who because of their particular circumstances are vulnerable to undue influence. However, this prohibition does not preclude (1) attempting to implement appropriate collateral contacts for the purpose of benefiting an already engaged therapy client/patient or (2) providing disaster or community outreach services.

6. Record Keeping and Fees

6.01 *Documentation of Professional and Scientific Work and Maintenance of Records*. Psychologists create, and to the extent the records are under their control, maintain, disseminate, store, retain, and dispose of records and data relating to their professional and scientific work in order to (1) facilitate provision of services later by them or by other professionals, (2) allow for replication of research design and analyses, (3) meet institutional requirements, (4) ensure accuracy of billing and payments, and (5) ensure compliance with law. (See also Standard 4.01, Maintaining Confidentiality.)

6.02 *Maintenance, Dissemination, and Disposal of Confidential Records of Professional and Scientific Work*. (a) Psychologists maintain confidentiality in creating, storing, accessing, transferring, and disposing of records under their control, whether these are written, automated, or in any other medium. (See also Standards 4.01, Maintaining Confidentiality, and 6.01, Documentation of Professional and Scientific Work and Maintenance of Records.)

(b) If confidential information concerning recipients of psychological services is entered into databases or systems of records available to persons whose access has not been consented to by the recipient, psychologists use coding or other techniques to avoid the inclusion of personal identifiers.

(c) Psychologists make plans in advance to facilitate the appropriate transfer and to protect the confidentiality of records and data in the event of psychologists' withdrawal from positions or practice. (See also Standards 3.12, Interruption of Psychological Services, and 10.09, Interruption of Therapy.)

6.03 *Withholding Records for Nonpayment*. Psychologists may not withhold records under their control that are requested and needed for a client's/patient's emergency treatment solely because payment has not been received.

6.04 *Fees and Financial Arrangements*. (a) As early as is feasible in a professional or scientific relationship, psychologists and recipients of psychological services reach an agreement specifying compensation and billing arrangements.

(b) Psychologists' fee practices are consistent with law.

(c) Psychologists do not misrepresent their fees.

(d) If limitations to services can be anticipated because of limitations in financing, this is discussed with the recipient of services as early as is feasible. (See also Standards 10.09, Interruption of Therapy, and 10.10, Terminating Therapy.)

(e) If the recipient of services does not pay for services as agreed, and if psychologists intend to use collection agencies or legal measures to collect the fees, psychologists first inform the person that such measures will be taken and provide that person an opportunity to make prompt payment. (See also Standards 4.05, Disclosures; 6.03, Withholding Records for Non-payment; and 10.01, Informed Consent to Therapy.)

6.05 *Barter With Clients/Patients.* Barter is the acceptance of goods, services, or other nonmonetary remuneration from clients/patients in return for psychological services. Psychologists may barter only if (1) it is not clinically contraindicated, and (2) the resulting arrangement is not exploitative. (See also Standards 3.05, Multiple Relationships, and 6.04, Fees and Financial Arrangements.)

6.06 *Accuracy in Reports to Payors and Funding Sources.* In their reports to payors for services or sources of research funding, psychologists take reasonable steps to ensure the accurate reporting of the nature of the service provided or research conducted, the fees, charges, or payments, and where applicable, the identity of the provider, the findings, and the diagnosis. (See also Standards 4.01, Maintaining Confidentiality; 4.04, Minimizing Intrusions on Privacy; and 4.05, Disclosures.)

6.07 *Referrals and Fees.* When psychologists pay, receive payment from, or divide fees with another professional, other than in an employer–employee relationship, the payment to each is based on the services provided (clinical, consultative, administrative, or other) and is not based on the referral itself. (See also Standard 3.09, Cooperation With Other Professionals.)

7. Education and Training

7.01 *Design of Education and Training Programs.* Psychologists responsible for education and training programs take reasonable steps to ensure that the programs are designed to provide the appropriate knowledge and proper experiences, and to meet the requirements for licensure, certification, or other goals for which claims are made by the program. (See also Standard 5.03, Descriptions of Workshops and Non-Degree-Granting Educational Programs.)

7.02 *Descriptions of Education and Training Programs.* Psychologists responsible for education and training programs take reasonable steps to ensure that there is a current and accurate description of the program content (including participation in required course- or program-related counseling, psychotherapy, experiential groups, consulting projects, or community service), training goals and objectives, stipends and benefits, and requirements that must be met for satisfactory completion of the program. This information must be made readily available to all interested parties.

7.03 Accuracy in Teaching. (a) Psychologists take reasonable steps to ensure that course syllabi are accurate regarding the subject matter to be covered, bases for evaluating progress, and the nature of course experiences. This standard does not preclude an instructor from modifying course content or requirements when the instructor considers it pedagogically necessary or desirable, so long as students are made aware of these modifications in a manner that enables them to fulfill course requirements. (See also Standard 5.01, Avoidance of False or Deceptive Statements.)

(b) When engaged in teaching or training, psychologists present psychological information accurately. (See also Standard 2.03, Maintaining Competence.)

7.04 Student Disclosure of Personal Information. Psychologists do not require students or supervisees to disclose personal information in course- or program-related activities, either orally or in writing, regarding sexual history, history of abuse and neglect, psychological treatment, and relationships with parents, peers, and spouses or significant others except if (1) the program or training facility has clearly identified this requirement in its admissions and program materials or (2) the information is necessary to evaluate or obtain assistance for students whose personal problems could reasonably be judged to be preventing them from performing their training- or professionally related activities in a competent manner or posing a threat to the students or others.

7.05 Mandatory Individual or Group Therapy. (a) When individual or group therapy is a program or course requirement, psychologists responsible for that program allow students in undergraduate and graduate programs the option of selecting such therapy from practitioners unaffiliated with the program. (See also Standard 7.02, Descriptions of Education and Training Programs.)

(b) Faculty who are or are likely to be responsible for evaluating students' academic performance do not themselves provide that therapy. (See also Standard 3.05, Multiple Relationships.)

7.06 Assessing Student and Supervisee Performance. (a) In academic and supervisory relationships, psychologists establish a timely and specific process for providing feedback to students and supervisees. Information regarding the process is provided to the student at the beginning of supervision.

(b) Psychologists evaluate students and supervisees on the basis of their actual performance on relevant and established program requirements.

7.07 Sexual Relationships With Students and Supervisees. Psychologists do not engage in sexual relationships with students or supervisees who are in their department, agency, or training center or over whom psychologists have or are likely to have evaluative authority. (See also Standard 3.05, Multiple Relationships.)

8. Research and Publication

8.01 *Institutional Approval.* When institutional approval is required, psychologists provide accurate information about their research proposals and obtain approval prior to conducting the research. They conduct the research in accordance with the approved research protocol.

8.02 *Informed Consent to Research.* (a) When obtaining informed consent as required in Standard 3.10, Informed Consent, psychologists inform participants about (1) the purpose of the research, expected duration, and procedures; (2) their right to decline to participate and to withdraw from the research once participation has begun; (3) the foreseeable consequences of declining or withdrawing; (4) reasonably foreseeable factors that may be expected to influence their willingness to participate such as potential risks, discomfort, or adverse effects; (5) any prospective research benefits; (6) limits of confidentiality; (7) incentives for participation; and (8) whom to contact for questions about the research and research participants' rights. They provide opportunity for the prospective participants to ask questions and receive answers. (See also Standards 8.03, Informed Consent for Recording Voices and Images in Research; 8.05, Dispensing With Informed Consent for Research; and 8.07, Deception in Research.)

(b) Psychologists conducting intervention research involving the use of experimental treatments clarify to participants at the outset of the research (1) the experimental nature of the treatment; (2) the services that will or will not be available to the control group(s) if appropriate; (3) the means by which assignment to treatment and control groups will be made; (4) available treatment alternatives if an individual does not wish to participate in the research or wishes to withdraw once a study has begun; and (5) compensation for or monetary costs of participating including, if appropriate, whether reimbursement from the participant or a third-party payor will be sought. (See also Standard 8.02a, Informed Consent to Research.)

8.03 *Informed Consent for Recording Voices and Images in Research.* Psychologists obtain informed consent from research participants prior to recording their voices or images for data collection unless (1) the research consists solely of naturalistic observations in public places, and it is not anticipated that the recording will be used in a manner that could cause personal identification or harm, or (2) the research design includes deception, and consent for the use of the recording is obtained during debriefing. (See also Standard 8.07, Deception in Research.)

8.04 Client/Patient, Student, and Subordinate Research Participants.
(a) When psychologists conduct research with clients/patients, students, or subordinates as participants, psychologists take steps to protect the prospective participants from adverse consequences of declining or withdrawing from participation.

(b) When research participation is a course requirement or an opportunity for extra credit, the prospective participant is given the choice of equitable alternative activities.

8.05 Dispensing With Informed Consent for Research. Psychologists may dispense with informed consent only (1) where research would not reasonably be assumed to create distress or harm and involves (a) the study of normal educational practices, curricula, or classroom management methods conducted in educational settings; (b) only anonymous questionnaires, naturalistic observations, or archival research for which disclosure of responses would not place participants at risk of criminal or civil liability or damage their financial standing, employability, or reputation, and confidentiality is protected; or (c) the study of factors related to job or organization effectiveness conducted in organizational settings for which there is no risk to participants' employability, and confidentiality is protected or (2) where otherwise permitted by law or federal or institutional regulations.

8.06 Offering Inducements for Research Participation. (a) Psychologists make reasonable efforts to avoid offering excessive or inappropriate financial or other inducements for research participation when such inducements are likely to coerce participation.

(b) When offering professional services as an inducement for research participation, psychologists clarify the nature of the services, as well as the risks, obligations, and limitations. (See also Standard 6.05, Barter With Clients/Patients.)

8.07 Deception in Research. (a) Psychologists do not conduct a study involving deception unless they have determined that the use of deceptive techniques is justified by the study's significant prospective scientific, educational, or applied value and that effective nondeceptive alternative procedures are not feasible.

(b) Psychologists do not deceive prospective participants about research that is reasonably expected to cause physical pain or severe emotional distress.

(c) Psychologists explain any deception that is an integral feature of the design and conduct of an experiment to participants as early as is feasible, preferably at the conclusion of their participation, but no later than at the conclusion of the data collection, and permit participants to withdraw their data. (See also Standard 8.08, Debriefing.)

8.08 Debriefing. (a) Psychologists provide a prompt opportunity for participants to obtain appropriate information about the nature, results, and conclusions of the research, and they take reasonable steps to correct any misconceptions that participants may have of which the psychologists are aware.

(b) If scientific or humane values justify delaying or withholding this information, psychologists take reasonable measures to reduce the risk of harm.

(c) When psychologists become aware that research procedures have harmed a participant, they take reasonable steps to minimize the harm.

8.09 Humane Care and Use of Animals in Research. (a) Psychologists acquire, care for, use, and dispose of animals in compliance with current federal, state, and local laws and regulations, and with professional standards.

(b) Psychologists trained in research methods and experienced in the care of laboratory animals supervise all procedures involving animals and are responsible for ensuring appropriate consideration of their comfort, health, and humane treatment.

(c) Psychologists ensure that all individuals under their supervision who are using animals have received instruction in research methods and in the care, maintenance, and handling of the species being used, to the extent appropriate to their role. (See also Standard 2.05, Delegation of Work to Others.)

(d) Psychologists make reasonable efforts to minimize the discomfort, infection, illness, and pain of animal subjects.

(e) Psychologists use a procedure subjecting animals to pain, stress, or privation only when an alternative procedure is unavailable and the goal is justified by its prospective scientific, educational, or applied value.

(f) Psychologists perform surgical procedures under appropriate anesthesia and follow techniques to avoid infection and minimize pain during and after surgery.

(g) When it is appropriate that an animal's life be terminated, psychologists proceed rapidly, with an effort to minimize pain and in accordance with accepted procedures.

8.10 Reporting Research Results. (a) Psychologists do not fabricate data. (See also Standard 5.01a, Avoidance of False or Deceptive Statements.)

(b) If psychologists discover significant errors in their published data, they take reasonable steps to correct such errors in a correction, retraction, erratum, or other appropriate publication means.

8.11 Plagiarism. Psychologists do not present portions of another's work or data as their own, even if the other work or data source is cited occasionally.

8.12 Publication Credit. (a) Psychologists take responsibility and credit, including authorship credit, only for work they have actually performed or to which they have substantially contributed. (See also Standard 8.12b, Publication Credit.)

(b) Principal authorship and other publication credits accurately reflect the relative scientific or professional contributions of the individuals involved, regardless of their relative status. Mere possession of an institutional position, such as department chair, does not justify authorship credit. Minor contributions to the research or to the writing for publications are acknowledged appropriately, such as in footnotes or in an introductory statement.

(c) Except under exceptional circumstances, a student is listed as principal author on any multiple-authored article that is substantially based on the student's doctoral dissertation. Faculty advisors discuss publication credit with students as early as feasible and throughout the research and publication process as appropriate. (See also Standard 8.12b, Publication Credit.)

8.13 Duplicate Publication of Data. Psychologists do not publish, as original data, data that have been previously published. This does not preclude republishing data when they are accompanied by proper acknowledgment.

8.14 Sharing Research Data for Verification. (a) After research results are published, psychologists do not withhold the data on which their conclusions are based from other competent professionals who seek to verify the substantive claims through reanalysis and who intend to use such data only for that purpose, provided that the confidentiality of the participants can be protected and unless legal rights concerning proprietary data preclude their release. This does not preclude psychologists from requiring that such individuals or groups be responsible for costs associated with the provision of such information.

(b) Psychologists who request data from other psychologists to verify the substantive claims through reanalysis may use shared data only for the declared purpose. Requesting psychologists obtain prior written agreement for all other uses of the data.

8.15 Reviewers. Psychologists who review material submitted for presentation, publication, grant, or research proposal review respect the confidentiality of and the proprietary rights in such information of those who submitted it.

9. Assessment

9.01 Bases for Assessments. (a) Psychologists base the opinions contained in their recommendations, reports, and diagnostic or evaluative statements, including forensic testimony, on information and techniques sufficient to substantiate their findings. (See also Standard 2.04, Bases for Scientific and Professional Judgments.)

(b) Except as noted in 9.01c, psychologists provide opinions of the psychological characteristics of individuals only after they have conducted an examination of the individuals adequate to support their statements or conclusions. When, despite reasonable efforts, such an examination is not practical, psychologists document the efforts they made and the result of those efforts, clarify the probable impact of their limited information on the reliability and validity of their opinions, and appropriately limit the nature and extent of their conclusions or recommendations. (See also Standards 2.01, Boundaries of Competence, and 9.06, Interpreting Assessment Results.)

(c) When psychologists conduct a record review or provide consultation or supervision and an individual examination is not warranted or necessary for the opinion, psychologists explain this and the sources of information on which they based their conclusions and recommendations.

9.02 *Use of Assessments.* (a) Psychologists administer, adapt, score, interpret, or use assessment techniques, interviews, tests, or instruments in a manner and for purposes that are appropriate in light of the research on or evidence of the usefulness and proper application of the techniques.

(b) Psychologists use assessment instruments whose validity and reliability have been established for use with members of the population tested. When such validity or reliability has not been established, psychologists describe the strengths and limitations of test results and interpretation.

(c) Psychologists use assessment methods that are appropriate to an individual's language preference and competence, unless the use of an alternative language is relevant to the assessment issues.

9.03 *Informed Consent in Assessments.* (a) Psychologists obtain informed consent for assessments, evaluations, or diagnostic services, as described in Standard 3.10, Informed Consent, except when (1) testing is mandated by law or governmental regulations; (2) informed consent is implied because testing is conducted as a routine educational, institutional, or organizational activity (e.g., when participants voluntarily agree to assessment when applying for a job); or (3) one purpose of the testing is to evaluate decisional capacity. Informed consent includes an explanation of the nature and purpose of the assessment, fees, involvement of third parties, and limits of confidentiality and sufficient opportunity for the client/patient to ask questions and receive answers.

(b) Psychologists inform persons with questionable capacity to consent or for whom testing is mandated by law or governmental regulations about the nature and purpose of the proposed assessment services, using language that is reasonably understandable to the person being assessed.

(c) Psychologists using the services of an interpreter obtain informed consent from the client/patient to use that interpreter, ensure that confidentiality of test results and test security are maintained, and include in their recommendations, reports, and diagnostic or evaluative statements, including forensic testimony, discussion of any limitations on the data obtained. (See also Standards 2.05, Delegation of Work to Others; 4.01, Maintaining Confidentiality; 9.01, Bases for Assessments; 9.06, Interpreting Assessment Results; and 9.07, Assessment by Unqualified Persons.)

9.04 *Release of Test Data.* (a) The term *test data* refers to raw and scaled scores, client/patient responses to test questions or stimuli, and psychologists' notes and recordings concerning client/patient statements and behavior during an examination. Those portions of test materials that include client/patient responses are included in the definition of *test data*. Pursuant to a client/patient release, psychologists provide test data to the client/patient or other persons identified in the release. Psychologists may refrain from releasing test data to protect a client/patient or others from substantial harm or misuse or misrepresentation of the data or the test, recognizing that in many instances release of confidential information under these circumstances is regulated by law. (See also Standard 9.11, Maintaining Test Security.)

(b) In the absence of a client/patient release, psychologists provide test data only as required by law or court order.

9.05 *Test Construction.* Psychologists who develop tests and other assessment techniques use appropriate psychometric procedures and current scientific or professional knowledge for test design, standardization, validation, reduction or elimination of bias, and recommendations for use.

9.06 *Interpreting Assessment Results.* When interpreting assessment results, including automated interpretations, psychologists take into account the purpose of the assessment as well as the various test factors, test-taking abilities, and other characteristics of the person being assessed, such as situational, personal, linguistic, and cultural differences, that might affect psychologists' judgments or reduce the accuracy of their interpretations. They indicate any significant limitations of their interpretations. (See also Standards 2.01b and 2.01c, Boundaries of Competence, and 3.01, Unfair Discrimination.)

9.07 *Assessment by Unqualified Persons.* Psychologists do not promote the use of psychological assessment techniques by unqualified persons, except when such use is conducted for training purposes with appropriate supervision. (See also Standard 2.05, Delegation of Work to Others.)

9.08 *Obsolete Tests and Outdated Test Results.* (a) Psychologists do not base their assessment or intervention decisions or recommendations on data or test results that are outdated for the current purpose.

(b) Psychologists do not base such decisions or recommendations on tests and measures that are obsolete and not useful for the current purpose.

9.09 *Test Scoring and Interpretation Services.* (a) Psychologists who offer assessment or scoring services to other professionals accurately describe the purpose, norms, validity, reliability, and applications of the procedures and any special qualifications applicable to their use.

(b) Psychologists select scoring and interpretation services (including automated services) on the basis of evidence of the validity of the program and procedures as well as on other appropriate considerations. (See also Standard 2.01b and 2.01c, Boundaries of Competence.)

(c) Psychologists retain responsibility for the appropriate application, interpretation, and use of assessment instruments, whether they score and interpret such tests themselves or use automated or other services.

9.10 *Explaining Assessment Results.* Regardless of whether the scoring and interpretation are done by psychologists, by employees or assistants, or by automated or other outside services, psychologists take reasonable steps to ensure that explanations of results are given to the individual or designated representative unless the nature of the relationship precludes provision of an explanation of results (such as in some organizational consulting, preemployment or security screenings, and forensic evaluations), and this fact has been clearly explained to the person being assessed in advance.

9.11 *Maintaining Test Security.* The term *test materials* refers to manuals, instruments, protocols, and test questions or stimuli and does not include *test data* as defined in Standard 9.04, Release of Test Data. Psychologists make reasonable efforts to maintain the integrity and security of test materials and other assessment techniques consistent with law and contractual obligations, and in a manner that permits adherence to this Ethics Code.

10. Therapy

10.01 *Informed Consent to Therapy.* (a) When obtaining informed consent to therapy as required in Standard 3.10, Informed Consent, psychologists inform clients/patients as early as is feasible in the therapeutic relationship about the nature and anticipated course of therapy, fees, involvement of third parties, and limits of confidentiality and provide sufficient opportunity for the client/patient to ask questions and receive answers. (See also Standards 4.02, Discussing the Limits of Confidentiality, and 6.04, Fees and Financial Arrangements.)

(b) When obtaining informed consent for treatment for which generally recognized techniques and procedures have not been established, psychologists inform their clients/patients of the developing nature of the treatment, the potential risks involved, alternative treatments that may be available, and the voluntary nature of their participation. (See also Standards 2.01d, Boundaries of Competence, and 3.10, Informed Consent.)

(c) When the therapist is a trainee and the legal responsibility for the treatment provided resides with the supervisor, the client/patient, as part of the informed consent procedure, is informed that the therapist is in training and is being supervised and is given the name of the supervisor.

10.02 Therapy Involving Couples or Families. (a) When psychologists agree to provide services to several persons who have a relationship (such as spouses, significant others, or parents and children), they take reasonable steps to clarify at the outset (1) which of the individuals are clients/patients and (2) the relationship the psychologist will have with each person. This clarification includes the psychologist's role and the probable uses of the services provided or the information obtained. (See also Standard 4.02, Discussing the Limits of Confidentiality.)

(b) If it becomes apparent that psychologists may be called on to perform potentially conflicting roles (such as family therapist and then witness for one party in divorce proceedings), psychologists take reasonable steps to clarify and modify, or withdraw from, roles appropriately. (See also Standard 3.05c, Multiple Relationships.)

10.03 Group Therapy. When psychologists provide services to several persons in a group setting, they describe at the outset the roles and responsibilities of all parties and the limits of confidentiality.

10.04 Providing Therapy to Those Served by Others. In deciding whether to offer or provide services to those already receiving mental health services elsewhere, psychologists carefully consider the treatment issues and the potential client's/patient's welfare. Psychologists discuss these issues with the client/patient or another legally authorized person on behalf of the client/patient in order to minimize the risk of confusion and conflict, consult with the other service providers when appropriate, and proceed with caution and sensitivity to the therapeutic issues.

10.05 Sexual Intimacies With Current Therapy Clients/Patients. Psychologists do not engage in sexual intimacies with current therapy clients/patients.

10.06 Sexual Intimacies With Relatives or Significant Others of Current Therapy Clients/Patients. Psychologists do not engage in sexual intimacies with individuals they know to be close relatives, guardians, or significant others of current clients/patients. Psychologists do not terminate therapy to circumvent this standard.

10.07 Therapy With Former Sexual Partners. Psychologists do not accept as therapy clients/patients persons with whom they have engaged in sexual intimacies.

10.08 Sexual Intimacies With Former Therapy Clients/Patients. (a) Psychologists do not engage in sexual intimacies with former clients/patients for at least two years after cessation or termination of therapy.

(b) Psychologists do not engage in sexual intimacies with former clients/patients even after a two-year interval except in the most unusual circumstances. Psychologists who engage in such activity after the two years following cessation or termination of therapy and of having no sexual contact with the former client/patient bear the burden of demonstrating that there has been no exploitation, in light of all relevant factors, including (1) the amount of time that has passed since therapy terminated; (2) the nature, duration, and intensity of the therapy; (3) the circumstances of termination; (4) the client's/patient's personal history; (5) the client's/patient's current mental status; (6) the likelihood of adverse impact on the client/patient; and (7) any statements or actions made by the therapist during the course of therapy suggesting or inviting the possibility of a posttermination sexual or romantic relationship with the client/patient. (See also Standard 3.05, Multiple Relationships.)

10.09 *Interruption of Therapy.* When entering into employment or contractual relationships, psychologists make reasonable efforts to provide for orderly and appropriate resolution of responsibility for client/patient care in the event that the employment or contractual relationship ends, with paramount consideration given to the welfare of the client/patient. (See also Standard 3.12, Interruption of Psychological Services.)

10.10 *Terminating Therapy.* (a) Psychologists terminate therapy when it becomes reasonably clear that the client/patient no longer needs the service, is not likely to benefit, or is being harmed by continued service.

(b) Psychologists may terminate therapy when threatened or otherwise endangered by the client/patient or another person with whom the client/patient has a relationship.

(c) Except where precluded by the actions of clients/patients or third-party payors, prior to termination psychologists provide pretermination counseling and suggest alternative service providers as appropriate.

The APA has previously published its Ethics Code as follows:

American Psychological Association. (1953). *Ethical standards of psychologists.* Washington, DC: Author.

American Psychological Association. (1959). Ethical standards of psychologists. *American Psychologist, 14,* 279–282.

American Psychological Association. (1963). Ethical standards of psychologists. *American Psychologist, 18,* 56–60.

American Psychological Association. (1968). Ethical standards of psychologists. *American Psychologist, 23,* 357–361.

American Psychological Association. (1977, March). Ethical standards of psychologists. *APA Monitor,* 22–23.

American Psychological Association. (1979). *Ethical standards of psychologists.* Washington, DC: Author.

American Psychological Association. (1981). Ethical principles of psychologists. *American Psychologist, 36,* 633–638.

American Psychological Association. (1990). Ethical principles of psychologists (Amended June 2, 1989). *American Psychologist, 45*, 390–395.

American Psychological Association. (1992). Ethical principles of psychologists and code of conduct. *American Psychologist, 47*, 1597–1611.

Request copies of the APA's "Ethical Principles of Psychologists and Code of Conduct" from the APA Order Department, 750 First Street, NE, Washington, DC 20002-4242, or phone (202) 336-5510.

REFERENCES

Adelman Steel Corp v. Winter, 610 So.2d 494; Fla. 1st DCA 1992.

American Academy of Child and Adolescent Psychiatry. (1997a). Practice parameters for child custody evaluation. *Journal of the American Academy of Child & Adolescent Psychiatry, 36*(Suppl. 10), 57–68.

American Academy of Child and Adolescent Psychiatry. (1997b). Practice parameters for the forensic evaluation of children and adolescents who may have been physically or sexually abused. *Journal of the American Academy of Child & Adolescent Psychiatry, 36*(Suppl. 10), 37–56.

American Academy of Clinical Neuropsychology. (1999). Policy on the use of non-doctoral-level personnel in conducting clinical neuropsychological evaluations. *The Clinical Neuropsychologists, 13,* 385.

American Academy of Clinical Neuropsychology. (2001). Policy statement on the presence of third party observers in neuropsychological assessments. *The Clinical Neuropsychologist, 15,* 433–439.

American Academy of Clinical Neuropsychology. (2003). Official position of the American Academy of Clinical Neuropsychology on ethical complaints made against clinical neuropsychologists during adversarial proceedings. *The Clinical Neuropsychologist, 17,* 443–445.

American Academy of Pediatrics, Committee on Child Abuse and Neglect. (1999). Guidelines for the evaluation of sexual abuse of children: Subject review. *Pediatrics, 103,* 186–191.

American Academy of Psychiatry and the Law. (1995). *Ethical guidelines for the practice of forensic psychiatry.* Bloomfield, CT: Author.

American Bar Association. (1989). *Criminal justice mental health standards.* Washington, DC: Author. Retrieved March 31, 2004, from http://www.abanet.org/crimjust/standards/mentalhealth_blk.html

American Educational Research Association, American Psychological Association, & National Council on Measurement in Education. (1999). *Standards for educational and psychological testing.* Washington, DC: Author.

American Medical Association. (1993a). *The insanity defense in criminal trials and limitations of psychiatric testimony.* Washington, DC: Author. Retrieved May 19, 2005, from http://www.ama-assn.org/

American Medical Association. (1993b). *Rape victim services.* Washington, DC: Author. Retrieved May 19, 2005, from http://www.ama-assn.org/

American Medical Association. (1997). *Bonding programs for women prisoners and their newborn children.* Washington, DC: Author. Retrieved May 19, 2005, from http://www.ama-assn.org/

American Medical Association. (1998a). *AMA–ABA statement on interprofessional relations for physicians and attorneys.* Washington, DC: Author. Retrieved May 19, 2005, from http://www.ama-assn.org/

American Medical Association. (1998b). *Guidelines for due process*. Washington, DC: Author. Retrieved May 19, 2005, from http://www.ama-assn.org/

American Medical Association. (1999a). *AMA code of ethics: E-5.09. Confidentiality industry-employed physicians and independent medical examiners*. Retrieved May 19, 2005, from http://www.ama-assn.org/ama/pub/category/8363.html

American Medical Association. (1999b). *AMA code of ethics: E-10.03. Patient–physician relationships in the context of work-related and independent medical examinations*. Retrieved May 19, 2005, from http://www.ama-assn.org/ama/pub/category/8326.html

American Medical Association. (2000a). *Guidelines for expert witness*. Retrieved May 19, 2005, from http://www.ama-assn.org/

American Medical Association. (2000b). *Peer review and medical expert witness testimony*. Retrieved May 19, 2005, from http://www.ama-assn.org/

American Medical Association. (2000c). *Prison-based treatment programs for drug abuse*. Retrieved May 19, 2005, from http://www.ama-assn.org/

American Medical Association. (2004a). *Expert witness affirmation*. Retrieved May 19, 2005, from http://www.ama-assn.org/

American Medical Association. (2004b). *Expert witness testimony*. Retrieved May 19, 2005, from http://www.ama-assn.org/

American Medical Association. (2004c). *Scientific status of refreshing recollection by the use of hypnosis*. Retrieved May 19, 2005, from http://www.ama-assn.org/

American Psychiatric Association. (1994). *Diagnostic and statistical manual of mental disorders* (4th ed.). Washington, DC: Author.

American Psychiatric Association. (1998). *Principles of medical ethics with annotations especially applicable to psychiatry*. Washington, DC: Author.

American Psychological Association. (1992). Ethical principles of psychologists and code of conduct. *American Psychologist, 47*, 1597–1611.

American Psychological Association. (1993). Record keeping guidelines. *American Psychologist, 48*, 984–986.

American Psychological Association. (1994). Guidelines for child custody evaluations in divorce proceedings. *American Psychologist, 49*, 677–680; also available at http://www.apa.org/practice/childcustody.html

American Psychological Association. (1999). Test security: Protecting the integrity of tests. *American Psychologist, 54*, 1078.

American Psychological Association. (2002). Ethical principles of psychologists and code of conduct. *American Psychologist, 57*, 1060–1073; also available at http://www.apa.org/ethics/code2002.html

Anderson, R. M., Jr., & Palozzi, A. M. (2002). Ethical issues in test construction, selection, and security. In S. S. Bush & M. L. Drexler (Eds.), *Ethical issues in clinical neuropsychology* (pp. 39–50). Lisse, the Netherlands: Swets & Zeitlinger.

Appelbaum, P. S., & Grisso, T. (1995). The MacArthur Treatment Competence Study: I. Mental illness and competence to consent to treatment. *Law and Human Behavior, 19*, 105–126.

Arkes, H. R. (1981). Impediments to accurate clinical judgment and variable ways to minimize their impact. *Journal of Consulting and Clinical Psychology, 49*, 323–330.

Arnoult, L. H., & Anderson, C. A. (1988). Identifying and reducing causal reasoning biases in clinical practice. In M. R. Leary & R. S. Miller (Eds.), *Social psychology and dysfunctional behavior: Origins, diagnosis, and treatment* (pp. 209–232). New York: Springer-Verlag.

Association of Family and Conciliation Courts. (1994). *Model standards of practice for child custody evaluation.* Milwaukee, WI: Author. Retrieved May 19, 2005, from http://www.afccnet.org/resources/resources_model_child.asp

Association of State and Provincial Psychology Boards. (2005). *ASPPB code of conduct* (Rev. ed.). Retrieved June 10, 2005, from http://www.asppb.org/publications/model/conduct.aspx

Bagby, R. M., Nicholson, R. A., Buis, T., Radovanvic, H., & Fidler, B. J. (1999). Defensive responding on the MMPI–2 in family custody and access evaluation. *Psychological Assessment, 11*, 24–28.

Barsky, A. E., & Gould, J. W. (2002). *Clinicians in court: A guide to subpoenas, depositions, testifying, and everything else you need to know.* New York: Guilford Press.

Bathurst, K., Gottfried, A. W., & Gottfried, A. E. (1997). Normative data for the MMPI–2 in child custody litigation. *Psychological Assessment, 9*, 205–211.

Beauchamp, T. L., & Childress, J. F. (2001). *Principles of biomedical ethics* (5th ed.). New York: Oxford University Press.

Behnke, S. H. (2003, November). Release of test data and APA's new Ethics Code. *Monitor on Psychology, 34*, 70–72.

Behnke, S. H., Perlin, M. L., & Bernstein, M. (2003). *The essentials of New York mental health law.* New York: Norton.

Bennett, B. E., Bryant, B. K., VandenBos, G. R., & Greenwood, A. (1990). *Professional liability and risk management.* Washington, DC: American Psychological Association.

Bieliauskas, L. A. (1999). The measurement of personality and emotional functioning. In J. J. Sweet (Ed.), *Forensic neuropsychology: Fundamentals and practice* (pp. 121–143). Lisse, the Netherlands: Swets & Zeitlinger.

Blase, J. J. (2003). Trained third-party presence during forensic neuropsychological evaluations. In A. M. Horton Jr. & L. C. Hartlage (Eds.), *Handbook of forensic neuropsychology* (pp. 369–382). New York: Springer Publishing Company.

Blau, T. H. (1998). *The psychologist as expert witness* (2nd ed.). New York: Wiley.

Bow, J. N., & Quinnell, F. A. (2001). Psychologists' current practices and procedures in child custody evaluations: Five years after the American Psychological Association Guidelines. *Professional Psychology: Research and Practice, 32*, 261–268.

Brigham, J. (1999). What is forensic psychology, anyway? *Law and Human Behavior, 23*, 273–298.

Brodsky, S. L. (1991). *Testifying in court: Guidelines and maxims for the expert witness.* Washington, DC: American Psychological Association.

Brodsky, S. L. (1999). *The expert expert witness: More maxims and guidelines for testifying in court.* Washington, DC: American Psychological Association.

Bush, S. S. (2004a). Introduction to Section 1: Differences between the 1992 and 2002 Ethics Codes: A brief overview. In S. S. Bush (Ed.), *A casebook of ethical challenges in neuropsychology* (pp. 1–8). New York: Psychology Press.

Bush, S. S. (2004b). Introduction to Section 2: Ethical challenges in forensic neuropsychology. In S. S. Bush (Ed.), *A casebook of ethical challenges in neuropsychology* (pp. 9–14). New York: Psychology Press.

Bush, S. S. (2004c). Introduction to Section 9: Ethical challenges with ethnically and culturally diverse populations in neuropsychology. In S. S. Bush (Ed.), *A casebook of ethical challenges in neuropsychology* (pp. 159–161). New York: Psychology Press.

Bush, S. S. (2004d). Introduction to Section 13: Ethical challenges in the determination of response validity in neuropsychology. In S. S. Bush (Ed.), *A casebook of ethical challenges in neuropsychology* (pp. 227–228). New York: Psychology Press.

Bush, S. S., & National Academy of Neuropsychology Policy & Planning Committee. (2005). Independent and court-ordered forensic neuropsychological examinations: Official statement of the National Academy of Neuropsychology. *Archives of Clinical Neuropsychology, 20,* 997–1007

Bush, S. S., Ruff, R., Troster, A., Barth, J., Koffler, S., Pliskin, N., et al. (2005). Symptom validity assessment: Practice issues and medical necessity. NAN position paper. *Archives of Clinical Neuropsychology, 20,* 419–426.

Butcher, J. N., Dahlstrom, W. G., Graham, J. R., Tellegen, A., & Kaemmer, B. (1989). *Minnesota Multiphasic Personality Inventory (MMPI–II) Manual for administration and scoring.* Minneapolis: University of Minnesota Press.

Canadian Psychological Association. (1991). *Canadian code of ethics for psychologists* (Rev. ed.). Ottawa, Ontario, Canada: Author.

Canadian Psychological Association. (2000). *Canadian code of ethics for psychologists* (3rd ed.). Ottawa, Ontario, Canada: Author.

Canadian Psychological Association. (2001). *Practice guidelines for providers of psychological services.* Ottawa, Ontario, Canada: Author.

Cantor, N., & Mischel, W. (1979). Prototypes in person perception. In L. Berkowitz (Ed.), *Advances in experimental and social psychology* (Vol. 9, pp. 4–52). New York: Academic Press.

Ceci, S. J., & Bruck, M. (1995). *Jeopardy in the courtroom: A scientific analysis of children's testimony.* Washington, DC: American Psychological Association.

Ceci, S. J., & Hembrooke, H. (Eds.). (1998). *Expert witnesses in child abuse cases: What can and should be said in court.* Washington, DC: American Psychological Association.

Committee on Ethical Guidelines for Forensic Psychologists. (1991). Specialty guidelines for forensic psychologists. *Law and Human Behavior, 15,* 655–665.

Committee on Professional Practice and Standards. (1999). Guidelines for psychological evaluations in child protection matters. *American Psychologist, 54,* 586–593; also available at http://www.apa.org/practice/childprotection.html

Connell, M. A. (2003). A psychobiographical approach to the evaluation for sentence mitigation. *The Journal of Psychiatry & Law, 31,* 319–354.

Connell, M. A., & Koocher, G. (2003). HIPAA and forensic practice. *American Psychology Law Society News, 23,* 16–19.

Constantinou, M., Ashendorf, L., & McCaffrey, R. J. (2002). When the third party observer of a neuropsychological evaluation is an audio-recorder. *The Clinical Neuropsychologist, 16,* 407–412.

Constantinou, M., & McCaffrey, R. J. (2003). The effects of third party observation: When the observer is a video camera. *Archives of Clinical Neuropsychology, 18,* 788–789.

Crown, B. M., Fingerhut, H. S., & Lowenthal, S. J. (2003). Conflicts of interest and other pitfalls for the expert witness. In A. M. Horton Jr. & L. C. Hartlage (Eds.), *Handbook of forensic neuropsychology* (pp. 383–421). New York: Springer Publishing Company.

Cunningham, M. D., & Reidy, T. J. (2001). A matter of life or death: Special considerations and heightened practice standards in capital sentencing evaluations. *Behavioral Sciences and the Law, 19,* 473–490.

Darley, J. M., & Gross, P. H. (1983). A hypothesis-confirming bias in labeling effects. *Journal of Personality and Social Psychology, 44,* 20–33.

Daubert v. Merrell Dow Pharmaceuticals, Inc., 509 U.S. 579 (1993).

Deidan, C., & Bush, S. S. (2002). Addressing perceived ethical violations by colleagues. In S. S. Bush & M. L. Drexler (Eds.), *Ethical issues in clinical neuropsychology* (pp. 281–305). Lisse, the Netherlands: Swets & Zeitlinger.

Denney, R. L. (2004). Ethical challenges in forensic neuropsychology, Section 1. In S. S. Bush (Ed.), *A casebook of ethical challenges in neuropsychology* (pp. 15–22). New York: Psychology Press.

Denney, R. L. (2005). Criminal forensic neuropsychology and assessment of competency. In G. J. Larrabee (Ed.), *Forensic neuropsychology: A scientific approach* (pp. 378–424). New York: Oxford University Press.

Denney, R. L., & Wynkoop, T. F. (2000). Clinical neuropsychology in the criminal forensic setting. *Journal of Head Trauma Rehabilitation, 15,* 804–828.

Faust, D. (1986). Research on human judgment and its application to clinical practice. *Professional Psychology: Research and Practice, 17,* 420–430.

Federal Rules of Evidence for the United States Courts and Magistrates. (1975–2000). St. Paul, MN: West Publishing Company.

Fischoff, B. (1982). Debiasing. In D. Kahneman, P. Slovic, & A. Tversky (Eds.), *Judgment under uncertainty: Heuristics and biases* (pp. 424–444). Cambridge, England: Cambridge University Press.

Fisher, C. B. (2003a). *Decoding the Ethics Code: A practical guide for psychologists.* Thousand Oaks, CA: Sage.

Fisher, C. B. (2003b, January/February). Test data standard most notable change in new APA ethics code. *The National Psychologist, 12,* 12–13.

Fisher, J. M., Johnson-Greene, D., & Barth, J. T. (2002). Evaluation, diagnosis, and interventions in neuropsychology in general and with special populations: An overview. In S. S. Bush & M. L. Drexler (Eds.), *Ethical issues in clinical neuropsychology* (pp. 3–22). Lisse, the Netherlands: Swets & Zeitlinger.

Frye v. United States, 293 F. Supp. 1013 (D.C. Cir. 1923).

Gavett, B. E., Lynch, J. K., & McCaffrey, R. J. (2003). Third party observers: The effect size is greater than you might think. *Archives of Clinical Neuropsychology, 18,* 789–790.

Goodman, K. W. (1998). Bioethics and health informatics: An introduction. In K. W. Goodman (Ed.), *Ethics, computing, and medicine: Informatics and the transformation of health care* (pp. 1–31). Cambridge, England: Cambridge University Press.

Green, R. G. (1983). Evaluation apprehension and the social facilitation/inhibition of learning. *Motivation and Emotion, 7,* 203–211.

Greenberg, L. R., & Gould, J. W. (2001). The treating expert: A hybrid role with firm boundaries. *Professional Psychology: Research and Practice, 32,* 469–478.

Greenberg, S., & Shuman, D. (1997). Irreconcilable conflict between therapeutic and forensic roles. *Professional Psychology: Research and Practice, 28,* 50–57.

Greiffenstein, M. F., Gola, T., & Baker, W. J. (1995). MMPI–2 validity scales versus domain specific measures in detection of factitious traumatic brain injury. *The Clinical Neuropsychologist, 9,* 230–240.

Grisso, T. (1990). Evolving guidelines for divorce/custody evaluations. *Family and Conciliation Courts Review, 28,* 35–41.

Grisso, T. (2003). *Evaluating competencies: Forensic assessments and instruments* (2nd ed.). New York: Kluwer Academic/Plenum Publishers.

Grisso, T., & Appelbaum, P. S. (1998a). *Assessing competence to consent to treatment: A guide for physicians and other health professionals.* London: Oxford University Press.

Grisso, T., & Appelbaum, P. S. (1998b). *MacArthur Competence Assessment Tool for Treatment (MacCAT–T).* Sarasota, FL: Professional Resource Press.

Grote, C. L. (2004). Ethical challenges in forensic neuropsychology, part II. In S. S. Bush (Ed.), *A casebook of ethical challenges in neuropsychology* (pp. 23–29). New York: Psychology Press

Grote, C. L., Lewin, J. L., Sweet, J. J., & van Gorp, W. G. (2000). Responses to perceived unethical practices in clinical neuropsychology: Ethical and legal considerations. *The Clinical Neuropsychologist, 14,* 119–134.

Guerin, B. (1986). Mere presence effects in humans: A review. *Journal of Experimental Social Psychology, 22,* 38–77.

Haas, L., & Malouf, J. (2002). *Keeping up the good work: A practitioner's guide to mental health ethics* (3rd ed.). Sarasota, FL: Professional Resource Press.

Halleck, S. L. (1980). Psychology and legal change: On the limits of factual jurisprudence. *Law and Human Behavior, 4*, 147–199.

Handelsman, M., Knapp, S., & Gottlieb, M. (2002). Positive ethics. In R. Snyder & S. Lopez (Eds.), *Handbook of positive psychology* (pp. 731–744). New York: Oxford University Press.

Hanson, S. L., Guenther, R., Kerkhoff, T. R., & Liss, M. (2000). Ethics: Historical foundations, basic principles, and contemporary issues. In R. G. Frank & T. R. Elliott (Eds.), *Handbook of rehabilitation psychology* (pp. 629–643). Washington, DC: American Psychological Association.

Hartlage, L. C. (2003). Neuropsychology in the courtroom. In A. M. Horton Jr. & L. C. Hartlage (Eds.), *Handbook of forensic neuropsychology* (pp. 315–333). New York: Springer Publishing Company.

Heilbrun, K. (1992). The role of psychological testing in forensic assessment. *Law and Human Behavior, 16*, 257–272.

Heilbrun, K. (1995). Child custody evaluation: Critically assessing mental health experts and psychological tests. *Family Law Quarterly, 29*, 63–78.

Heilbrun, K. (2001). *Principles of forensic mental health assessment.* New York: Kluwer Academic/Plenum Publishers.

Heilbrun, K., Warren, J., & Picarello, K. (2003). Third party information in forensic assessment. In A. Goldstein, (Ed.), *Handbook of forensic psychology* (pp. 69–86). Somerset, New Jersey: Wiley.

Iverson, G. L. (2000). Dual relationships in psycholegal evaluations: Treating psychologists service as expert witnesses. *American Journal of Forensic Psychology, 18*, 79–87.

Iverson, G. L. (2003). Detecting malingering in civil forensic evaluations. In A. M. Horton Jr. & L. C. Hartlage (Eds.), *Handbook of forensic neuropsychology* (pp. 137–177). New York: Springer Publishing Company.

Iverson, G. L., & Slick, D. J. (2003). Ethical issues associated with psychological and neuropsychological assessment of persons from different cultural and linguistic backgrounds. In I. Z. Schultz & D. O. Brady (Eds.), *Psychological injuries at trial* (pp. 2066–2087). Chicago: American Bar Association.

Johnson-Greene, D., & National Academy of Neuropsychology Policy & Planning Committee. (2003). *Informed consent in clinical neuropsychology practice: Official statement of the National Academy of Neuropsychology.* Retrieved January 16, 2004, from http://www.nanonline.org/paio/informed_consent.shtm

Kahneman, D., & Tversky, A. (1973). On the psychology of prediction. *Psychological Review, 80*, 237–251.

Kehrer, C. A., Sanchez, P. N., Habif, U. J., Rosenbaum, G. J., & Townes, B. D. (2000). Effects of a significant-other observer on neuropsychological test performance. *The Clinical Neuropsychologist, 14*, 67–71.

Kitchener, K. S. (2000). *Foundations of ethical practice, research, and teaching.* Mahwah, NJ: Erlbaum.

Knapp, S., & VandeCreek, L. (2003). *A guide to the 2002 revision of the American Psychological Association's Ethics Code.* Sarasota, FL: Professional Resource Press.

Koocher, G. P., & Keith-Spiegel, P. (1998). *Ethics in psychology: Professional standards and cases* (2nd ed.). New York: Oxford University Press.

Kuehnle, K. (1996). *Assessing allegations of child sexual abuse.* Sarasota, FL: Professional Resource Exchange.

Larrabee, G. J. (1998). Somatic malingering on the MMPI and MMPI–2 in litigating subjects. *The Clinical Neuropsychologist, 12,* 179–188.

Larrabee, G. J. (2003a). Detection of symptom exaggeration with the MMPI–2 in litigants with malingered neurocognitive dysfunction. *The Clinical Neuropsychologist, 17,* 54–68.

Larrabee, G. J. (2003b). Exaggerated MMPI–2 symptom report in personal injury litigants with malingered neurocognitive deficit. *Archives of Clinical Neuropsychology, 18,* 673–686.

Larrabee, G. J. (2005). Assessment of malingering. In G. J. Larrabee (Ed.), *Forensic neuropsychology: A scientific approach* (pp. 115–158). New York: Oxford University Press.

Lees-Haley, P. R. (1999). Commentary on Sweet and Moulthrop's debiasing procedures. *Journal of Forensic Neuropsychology, 1,* 43–47.

Lees-Haley, P. R., & Cohen, L. J. (1999). The neuropsychologist as expert witness: Toward credible science in the courtroom. In J. J. Sweet (Ed.), *Forensic neuropsychology: Fundamentals and practice* (pp. 443–468). Lisse, the Netherlands: Swets & Zeitlinger.

Lees-Haley, P. R., English, L. T., & Glenn, W. J. (1991). A Fake Bad Scale for the MMPI–2 for personal injury claimants. *Psychological Reports, 68,* 203–210.

Lezak, M. D. (1995). *Neuropsychological assessment* (3rd ed.). New York: Oxford University Press.

Lubet, S. (1999, Spring). Expert witnesses: Ethics and professionalism. *Georgetown Journal of Legal Ethics, 12,* 465–488.

Lynch, G. W. (1993). Foreword. In J. S. Wulach (Ed.), *Law & mental health professionals: New York* (p. 7). Washington, DC: American Psychological Association.

Lynch, J. K. (1997). The effect of observer's presence on neuropsychological test performance: A test of the social facilitation phenomenon. *Dissertation Abstracts International, 57,* 7230B.

Lynch, J. K. (2003). The effect of an observer on neuropsychological test performance following TBI. *Archives of Clinical Neuropsychology, 18,* 791.

Manly, J. J., & Jacobs, D. M. (2002). Future directions in neuropsychological assessment with African Americans. In F. R. Ferraro (Ed.), *Minority and cross-cultural aspects of neuropsychological assessment* (pp. 79–96). Lisse, the Netherlands: Swets & Zeitlinger.

Martelli, M. F., Bush, S. S., & Zasler, N. D. (2003). Identifying, avoiding, and addressing ethical misconduct in neuropsychological medicolegal practice. *International Journal of Forensic Psychology, 1*, 26–44.

Martindale, D. A., & Gould, J. W. (2004). The forensic model: Ethics and scientific methodology applied to custody evaluations. *Journal of Child Custody, 1*, 1–22.

McCaffrey, R. J., O'Bryant, S. E., Ashendorf, L., & Fisher, J. M. (2003). Correlations among the TOMM, Rey-15, and MMPI–2 validity scales in a sample of TBI litigants. *Journal of Forensic Neuropsychology, 3*, 45–54.

McLearen, A. M., Pietz, C. A., & Denney, R. L. (2004). Evaluation of psychological damages. In W. O'Donohue & E. Levensky (Eds.). *Handbook of forensic psychology* (pp. 267–299). San Diego, CA: Elsevier.

Melton, G. B., Petrila, J., Poythress, N. G., & Slobogin, C. (1997). *Psychological evaluations for the courts.* New York: Guilford Press.

Meyers, J. E., & Volbrecht, M. E. (2003). A validation of multiple malingering detection methods in a large clinical sample. *Archives of Clinical Neuropsychology, 18*, 261–276.

Mrad, D. (1996, September). *Criminal responsibility evaluations.* Paper presented at the Issues in Forensic Assessment Symposium, Federal Bureau of Prisons, Atlanta, GA.

Multi-Health Systems. (2003). *HIPAA position statement.* Retrieved April 5, 2004, from http://www.mhs.com

Nagy, T. F. (2000). *Ethics in plain English: An illustrative casebook for psychologists.* Washington, DC: American Psychological Association.

National Academy of Neuropsychology Policy & Planning Committee. (2000a). Presence of third party observers during neuropsychological testing: Official statement of the National Academy of Neuropsychology. *Archives of Clinical Neuropsychology, 15*, 379–380.

National Academy of Neuropsychology Policy & Planning Committee. (2000b). Test security: Official position statement of the National Academy of Neuropsychology. *Archives of Clinical Neuropsychology, 15*, 383–386.

National Academy of Neuropsychology Policy & Planning Committee. (2000c). The use of neuropsychology test technicians in clinical practice: Official statement of the National Academy of Neuropsychology. *Archives of Clinical Neuropsychology, 15*, 381–382.

National Academy of Neuropsychology Policy & Planning Committee. (2003). *Test Security: An update. Official statement of the National Academy of Neuropsychology.* Retrieved February 17, 2004, from http://nanonline.org/paio/security_update.shtm

Otto, R. K., Buffington-Vollum, J. K., & Edens, J. F. (2002). Child custody evaluation. In A. M. Goldstein (Ed.), *Comprehensive handbook of psychology: Vol. 11. Forensic psychology* (pp. 179–208). New York: Wiley.

Poole, D. A., & Lamb, M. E. (1998). *Investigative interviews of children: A guide for helping professionals.* Washington, DC: American Psychological Association.

Rapp, D. L., & Ferber, P. S. (2003). To release, or not to release raw test data, that is the question. In A. M. Horton Jr. & L. C. Hartlage (Eds.), *Handbook of forensic neuropsychology* (pp. 337–368). New York: Springer Publishing Company.

Rogers, R. (1997). Introduction. In R. Rogers (Ed.), *Clinical assessment of malingering and deception* (2nd ed., pp. 1–19). New York: Guilford Press.

Ross, L. (1977). The intuitive psychologist and his shortcomings: Distortions in the attribution process. In L. Berkowitz (Ed.), *Advances in experimental social psychology* (Vol. 10, pp. 173–220). New York: Academic Press.

Russell, A., Russell, G., & Midwinter, D. (1992). Observer influences on mothers and fathers: Self-reported influence during home observation. *Merill-Palmer Quarterly, 38,* 263–283.

Saks, M. J. (1990). Expert witnesses, nonexpert witnesses, and nonwitness experts. *Law and Human Behavior, 14,* 291–313.

Sales, B. D., & Miller, M. O. (1993). Editor's preface. In J. S. Wulach (Ed.), *Law & mental health professionals: New York* (pp. 1–5). Washington, DC: American Psychological Association.

Saywitz, K. J., & Snyder, L. (1996). Narrative elaboration: Test of a new procedure for interviewing children. *Journal of Consulting and Clinical Psychology, 64,* 1347–1357.

Sbordone, R. J., Rogers, M. L., Thomas, V. A., & de Armas, A. (2003). Forensic neuropsychological assessment in criminal cases. In A. M. Horton Jr. & L. C. Hartlage (Eds.), *Handbook of forensic neuropsychology* (pp. 471–503). New York: Springer Publishing Company.

Shapiro, D. L. (1991). *Forensic psychological assessment: An integrative approach.* Boston: Allyn & Bacon.

Shapiro, D. L. (1999). *Criminal responsibility evaluations.* Sarasota, FL: Professional Resource Press.

Shuman, D. W., & Greenberg, S. A. (1998, Winter). The role of ethical norms in the admissibility of expert testimony. *The Judge's Journal,* 5–9, 42.

Siegel, J. C. (1996). Traditional MMPI–2 validity indicators and initial presentation in custody evaluations. *American Journal of Forensic Psychology, 14,* 55–63.

Siegel, J. C., & Langford, J. S. (1998). MMPI–2 scales and suspected parental alienation syndrome. *American Journal of Forensic Psychology, 16,* 5–14.

Slick, D. J., & Iverson, G. L. (2003). Ethical issues in forensic neuropsychological assessment. In I. Z. Schultz & D. O. Brady (Eds.), *Psychological injuries at trial* (pp. 2014–2034). Chicago: American Bar Association.

Slick, D. J., Sherman, E. M. S., & Iverson, G. L. (1999). Diagnostic criteria for malingered neurocognitive dysfunction: Proposed standards for clinical practice and research. *The Clinical Neuropsychologist, 13,* 545–561.

Snyder, M., & Campbell, B. H. (1980). Testing hypotheses about people: The role of the hypothesis. *Personality and Social Psychology Bulletin, 6,* 421–426.

Stone, A. A. (1984). *Law, psychiatry, and morality*. Washington, DC: American Psychiatric Press.

Sweet, J. J. (1999). Malingering: Differential diagnosis. In J. J. Sweet (Ed.), *Forensic neuropsychology: Fundamentals and practice* (pp. 255–285). Lisse, the Netherlands: Swets & Zeitlinger.

Sweet, J. J., Grote, C., & van Gorp, W. G. (2002). Ethical issues in forensic neuropsychology. In S. S. Bush & M. Drexler (Eds.), *Ethical issues in clinical neuropsychology* (pp. 104–133). Lisse, the Netherlands: Swets & Zeitlinger.

Sweet, J. J., & Moulthrop, M. A. (1999a). Response to Lees-Haley's commentary: Debiasing techniques cannot be completely curative. *Journal of Forensic Neuropsychology, 1*, 49–57.

Sweet, J. J., & Moulthrop, M. A. (1999b). Self-examination questions as a means of identifying bias in adversarial assessments. *Journal of Forensic Neuropsychology, 1*, 73–88.

U.S. Department of Health and Human Services. (1996). *Public Law 104–191: Health Insurance Portability and Accountability Act of 1996*. Retrieved November 24, 2003, from http://www.hhs.gov/ocr/hipaa/

U.S. Security Insurance Co. v. Cimino, 754 So. 2d 697 (Fla. 2000).

Wainwright v. Greenfield, 474 U.S. 284, 106 S. Ct. 634 (1986).

Walker, L. A., & Shapiro, D. L. (2003). *Introduction to forensic psychology: Clinical and social psychological perspectives*. New York: Kluwer Academic/Plenum Publishers.

Wechsler, D. (1997). WAIS–III. *Administration and Scoring Manual*. San Antonio, TX: The Psychological Corporation.

Wells, G. L. (1982). Attribution and reconstructive memory. *Journal of Experimental and Social Psychology, 18*, 447–463.

Williams, C., Lees-Haley, P., & Djanogly, S. E. (1999). Clinical scrutiny of litigants' self-reports. *Professional Psychology: Research and Practice, 30*, 361–367.

Wynkoop, T. F., & Denney, R. L. (1999). Exaggeration of neuropsychological deficit in competency to stand trial. *Journal of Forensic Neuropsychology, 1*, 29–53.

AUTHOR INDEX

Green, R. G., 76, 77
Greenberg, L. R., 15
Greenberg, S., 12, 13, 14, 27, 114, 116, 126
Greenwood, A., 35
Grisso, T., 51, 61, 67, 74, 93, 119
Gross, P. H., 97
Grote, C. L., 53, 124
Guenther, R., 17
Guerin, B., 76

Haas, L., 28
Habif, U. J., 76
Halleck, S. L., 40
Handelsman, M., 27
Hanson, S. L., 17
Hartlage, L. C., 38
Heilbrun, K., 9, 10, 13, 14, 38, 40, 41, 42, 43, 45, 49, 50, 51, 52, 59, 60, 61, 62, 63, 67, 68, 70, 73, 74, 92, 93, 99, 114, 115, 119, 123, 127
Hembrooke, H., 65

Iverson, G. L., 12, 41, 68, 80, 81, 107

Jacobs, D. M., 80
Johnson-Greene, D., 12

Kahneman, D., 97
Kehrer, C. A., 76
Keith-Spiegel, P., 10, 28, 93
Kerkhoff, T. R., 17
Kitchener, K. S., 28
Knapp, S., 4, 19, 20, 22, 27, 28, 81
Koocher, G., 10, 26, 28, 93, 106, 109
Kuehnle, K., 65

Lamb, M. E., 65
Langford, J. S., 69
Larrabee, G. J., 67
Lees-Haley, P., 39, 65
Lewin, J. L., 124
Lezak, M. D., 70
Liss, M., 17
Lowenthal, S. J., 15

Lubet, S., 16
Lynch, G. W., 35
Lynch, J. K., 76

Malouf, J., 28
Manly, J. J., 80
Martelli, M. F., 16, 17, 99, 100, 124, 127
Martindale, D. A., 127
McCaffrey, R. J., 76
McLearen, A. M., 50, 51, 63
Melton, G. B., 10, 11, 13, 38, 41, 51, 63, 93, 99, 101
Midwinter, D., 76
Miller, M. O., 34
Mischel, W., 98
Moulthrop, M. A., 39, 72, 97, 99
Mrad, D., 63
Multi-Health Systems, 106

Nagy, T. F., 41, 128
National Academy of Neuropsychology Policy and Planning Committee, 60, 75, 77, 94, 100, 106, 109, 111, 116, 117
National Council on Measurement in Education, 60, 106
Nicholson, R. A., 69

Otto, R. K., 86, 134

Perlin, M. L., 10
Petrila, J., 10, 38, 51, 63, 93
Picarello, K., 49, 51, 127
Pietz, C. A., 50, 63
Poole, D. A., 65
Poythress, N. G., 10, 38, 51, 63, 93

Radovanvic, H., 69
Rapp, D. L., 103, 105, 107
Reidy, T. J., 82, 83
Rogers, M. L., 65
Rogers, R., 50
Rosenbaum, G. J., 76
Ross, L., 97
Russell, A., 76
Russell, G., 76

SUBJECT INDEX

Accuracy
  assumption of, 12
  in testimony, 114–115
Adelman Steel Corp. v. Winter (1992),
    78
Admissibility of evidence, 64, 74,
    126–127
Adversarial environment, 15–16
Adversarial system, 15, 17–19
Advocacy, in role of trial consultant, 40
Alliances, forensic psychologist and, 12,
    16
American Academy of Forensic
    Psychology, 23
American Bar Association, Criminal Jus-
    tice Mental Health Standards,
    10–12
American Board of Forensic Psychology,
    42
American Psychological Association. *See*
    APA Ethics Code
American Psychology—Law Society, 23,
    42
Anchoring, 98
APA Ethics Code, 5, 27
  avoidance of false or deceptive
    statements, 93, 115, 119
  bases for assessment, 69
  bases for judgments, 92
  confidentiality, 62
  ethical misconduct, 127–129, 136
  evaluation procedures, 63
  forensic application of, 19–22,
    19n2
  informed consent, 78
  misuse of psychologists' work, 115
  principles, 17, 30–31
  and professional competence, 41
  record reviews, 83–84
  release of test data, 104–108
  test security, 77
  use of assessments, 66, 76, 81
  use of deception in research, 73
Assent, 60–63

Assent form, use of, 62
Assessment, 21
  and ethnic/cultural diversity issues,
    81–82
  and informed consent, 20–21
Assessment instruments, 21
Assessment results, interpreting, 21
Association of State and Provincial Psy-
    chology Boards Code of Conduct,
    23, 129
Attorney. *See also* retaining-party/
    examiner relationship
Attorney, consultation with, 35, 108
Attorney tactics, and testimony, 115
Autonomy, principle of, 17, 30, 37, 49,
    53, 59, 64, 86–87, 107, 111
Availability heuristic, 97

Background, examinee's, investigation of,
    53
Background information
  collection of, 52–53
  and hypothesis testing, 98
  types of, 50–52
Barsky, A. E., 38
Bases for opinions, 50–52, 55
Beauchamp, T. L., 17–19, 30
Behavioral observations, 63–65
Behnke, S. H., 30, 35
Beliefs, personal, of forensic psychologist,
    32
Beneficence, principle of, 17, 19, 30, 41,
    92, 107, 110–111, 132
Bennett, B. E., 35
Bias. *See also* impartiality; objectivity;
    self-bias
  in collateral source information, 54
  financially motivated, 96, 116–117
  inferential, 96–99
  and modification of reports, 100
  risk of, 35, 39, 115, 124
  in test selection, 70
Bieliauskas, L. A., 65

De Armas, A., 65
Death penalty cases, 105
Debiasing procedures, 39
Deception, of examiner, 69, 73
Decision making, 93
    proposed model, 27–34
    surrogate, 59–60
Defamation of character, 129
Definitive statements, demand for, 93
Deidan, C., 99
Dialogue, with colleague, 125
Disclosure
    of raw test data, 103–109, 111
    of records, 108–112
    of test results in criminal cases,
        117–121
Djanogly, S. E., 65
Doctor–patient relationship, 60
Documentation, 35, 52, 91–92, 130
Due diligence, 52, 94–95
Due process, 95, 100–102

Emergencies, and professional
        competence, 41
Enticement, to ethical misconduct,
        139–140
Ethical decision making for forensic psy-
        chology, proposed model, 27–34
Ethical guidelines, for third-party
        observation, 76–77
Ethical misconduct, perceived, 124–137
Ethical problems, resolving, 20
    eight-step model, 27–34
Ethics and law, conflicts between, 27
Ethics Code, APA. See APA Ethics Code
Ethics codes, professional, 31. See also
        names of organizations
Ethics in forensic psychology, need for
        information on, 16
Ethnic diversity issues, 80–83
Evaluation, 11–12, 59
    of children, 79
    of criminal defendant, 64–65
    and ethnic/cultural diversity issues,
        80–83
    multisource, multimethod model,
        50–51, 54–56, 63
    third-party observation of, 75–80
Evaluation methods selection, legal
        considerations for, 74

Evaluation procedures and measures,
        63–73
Evaluator, clinical, 14
Evaluator, court-appointed, 14
Evidence, admissible, 64, 74, 126–127
Examinee statements, reproduction of,
        100–102
Examiner deception, 69, 73
Expert witness, 11–14, 13n1
    for defense, 14
    for plaintiff, 14
    for prosecution, 14
    and trial consultant, 40

Fact witness, 13, 13n1, 14
Family law, 10, 84–89, 130–137
Federal Rules of Evidence (FRE), 13n1,
        42, 50, 93, 103–104
Feedback
    concerning practice, 140
    in judicial referrals, 109
    provided to examinee, 63
Fee structure, 29, 42–44
Ferber, P. S., 105, 107
Financial arrangements, 29, 42–44
Financial incentive, 96, 116–117, 123–124
Fisher, C. B., 105–106
Florida Supreme Court, 78
Forensic evaluation services, 11–12
Forensic expert, role of, 38–40
Forensic psychologist, use of term, 10
Forensic psychology, 9, 42
    civil and criminal contexts, 10–15
Freedom of choice, 59
Frye v. United States (1923), 74, 91
Fundamental attribution error, 97–98

"General acceptance" standard, 74
Gould, J. W., 38
Green, R. G., 77
Greenberg, S., 116, 126
Greenwood, A., 35
Grisso, T., 93
Guidelines for Child Custody Evaluation
        in Divorce Proceedings, 86, 132

Health Insurance Portability and
        Accountability Act (HIPAA),
        23–26, 52, 105–106, 108–109

surreptitious, 64
third-party, 75–80
Observer
   involved, 77
   trained, 77–78
   uninvolved, 77
Opinion
   bases for, 50–52, 55
   limitations of, 93–94
Opinion data, 22
   misuse of, 13
Opponent, forensic psychologist
      perceived as, 16
Outcome, manipulation of, 70

Parenting issues, 84–89
Partisan expert, role of, 54–57
Peer review, 83–84, 91–92
Performance, affected by observation,
      75–76
Personal attack, 128–129
Personal injury law, 109–112
Personal responsibility, sense of, 18
Petrila, J., 93
Position statements, of professional
      associations, 31
Posttraumatic stress disorder (PTSD), 44–
      48, 117–121
Poythress, N. G., 93
Privacy rights, 49, 49n1, 64–65
Privilege, holder of, 126
Professional activities, and professional
      competence, 41
Professional guidelines, use of, 22–23
Psychological capacities, opinions on, 93
Psychological testing, 66–68
Psychologist–examinee relationship, 60,
      114
Psychotherapy notes, 108–109

Questionnaires, in information
      collection, 52

Rapp, D. L., 105, 107
Reactivity, 75–76
Reconstructive memory, 98–99
Recording devices, use of, 76
Record review, 22, 51, 55, 63, 83–84

Records
   destruction of, 110–112
   disclosure of, 108–109
   dual sets of, 108–109
   maintenance of, 117
Records, medical, inaccuracies in, 51
Referral question, responding to,
      94–96
Referrals, in personal injury litigation,
      44–48
Reidy, T. J., 82
Related issues, responding to, 94–96
Release, client–patient, 22
Relevance, of evidence, 50–51
Reliability, of evidence, 50
Reports, 99–103
   preliminary, 56–57, 102–103
Representative heuristic, 97
Reproduction, of examinee statements,
      100–102
Resolution of ethical problems, 20
   eight-step model, 27–34
Resources, ethical and legal, identifying
      and using, 30–32
Respectful receptivity, during
      examination, 12
Retaining party
   as client, 11
   and mandated measures, 74–75
Retaining-party/examiner relationship,
      37–40
Rey 15-Item Memory Test, 71
Rights
   to access medical records, 107
   to due process, 95, 100–102
   to have expert opinion derived from
      all relevant information, 49
   to privacy, 49, 49n1, 64–65
   to understand evaluation process and
      implications, 60
   to understand nature and purpose of
      evaluation, 59
   to withhold consent, 53
Risk-management strategies, application
      to forensic practice, 34–35
Rogers, M. L., 65
Rogers, R., 50
Role clarification, 38, 40, 45–48,
      113–114
Role conflicts, and use of preliminary
      reports, 102–103

VandeCreek, L., 5, 27–28, 81
VandenBos, G. R., 35
Video surveillance, 64

Wechsler Adult Intelligence Scale—
  Third Edition, 77

White papers, of professional
  associations, 31
Williams, C., 65
Witness. *See* expert witness; fact witness

ABOUT THE AUTHORS

Shane S. Bush, PhD, ABPP, ABPN, is in independent practice in Smith-town, New York. He is board certified in rehabilitation psychology by the American Board of Professional Psychology and is board certified in neuropsychology by the American Board of Professional Neuropsychology. He is a fellow of both the American Psychological Association, Division 40 (Clinical Neuropsychology), and the National Academy of Neuropsychology. He is an editorial board member of *The Clinical Neuropsychologist*, coediting the Ethical and Professional Issues section. He is also an editorial board member of the *Journal of Forensic Neuropsychology* and *Applied Neuropsychology*, for which he edited special issues on ethics. He is coeditor of the book *Ethical Issues in Clinical Neuropsychology*, editor of *A Casebook of Ethical Challenges in Neuropsychology*, coauthor of *Health Care Ethics for Psychologists: A Casebook*, and coeditor of *Geriatric Neuropsychology: Practice Essentials*. He has authored position papers on forensic matters for the National Academy of Neuropsychology and has presented on ethical issues at national conferences. He is a veteran of both the U.S. Marine Corps and U.S. Navy.

Mary A. Connell, EdD, ABPP, is in independent practice in Fort Worth, Texas. She is board certified in forensic psychology by the American Board of Professional Psychology. Primary areas of work are child custody evaluation, evaluations for sentence mitigation, and personal injury examinations. She is president of the American Academy of Forensic Psychology and is on the editorial board of the *Journal of Child Custody*. She provides workshops on parenting assessment for child custody/access matters and child protection matters and on ethics in forensic practice. She serves on the Committee on Professional Practice and Standards, a Board of Professional Affairs committee of the American Psychological Association. She has authored or coauthored articles on sexual abuse investigation in custody evaluation, focus of custody evaluation, interstate psychological practice considerations, evaluation for sentence mitigation in death penalty cases, and evaluation procedures in child custody matters.

Robert L. Denney, PsyD, ABPP, ABPN, has been a forensic psychologist and neuropsychologist at the U.S. Medical Center for Federal Prisoners in Springfield, Missouri, for over 14 years. He is also an associate professor and director of neuropsychology at the Forest Institute of Professional Psychology in Springfield. He is board certified in forensic psychology by the American Board of Professional Psychology and in neuropsychology by both the American Board of Professional Psychology and the American Board of Professional Neuropsychology. He is a fellow of the National Academy of Neuropsychology. Dr. Denney is on the editorial board of the *Journal of Forensic Neuropsychology*, for which he edited a special issue on negative response bias and criminal forensic neuropsychology. He is coeditor of *Detection of Response Bias in Forensic Neuropsychology* and coauthor of *Detection of Deception*. He has published in the scientific literature on such subjects as neuropsychological evaluation of criminal defendants, malingering, evaluating psychological damages, trauma and violence, ethical issues, and professional licensure. He has also presented throughout the United States on neurolitigation, the application of neuropsychology to criminal forensic matters, neuroanatomy, brain injury, malingering, and admissibility of scientific evidence. Opinions expressed here are those of the author and do not necessarily represent opinions of the Federal Bureau of Prisons or the Department of Justice.